Pedagogies of Woundedness

In the series *Dis/color*, edited by Cynthia Wu,
Julie Avril Minich, and Nirmala Erevelles

ALSO IN THIS SERIES:

Milo Obourn, *Disabled Futures: A Framework
for Radical Inclusion*

JAMES KYUNG-JIN LEE

Pedagogies of Woundedness

Illness, Memoir, and the Ends
of the Model Minority

TEMPLE UNIVERSITY PRESS
Philadelphia · Rome · Tokyo

TEMPLE UNIVERSITY PRESS
Philadelphia, Pennsylvania 19122
tupress.temple.edu

Library of Congress Cataloging-in-Publication Data

Names: Lee, James Kyung-Jin, author.
Title: Pedagogies of woundedness : illness, memoir, and the ends of the
  model minority / James Kyung-Jin Lee.
Description: Philadelphia : Temple University Press, 2022. | Series:
  Dis/color | Includes bibliographical references and index. | Summary:
  "Pedagogies of Woundedness wonders what happens when illness betrays
  fantasies of indefinite progress to those entrusted to live out this
  role framed by success: Asian Americans"—Provided by publisher.
Identifiers: LCCN 2021022985 (print) | LCCN 2021022986 (ebook) |
  ISBN 9781439921852 (cloth) | ISBN 9781439921869 (paperback) |
  ISBN 9781439921876 (pdf)
Subjects: LCSH: Asian Americans—Health and hygiene—Social aspects. |
  Asian Americans—Medical care—Social aspects. | Model minority
  stereotype—Health aspects. | Health and race—United States.
Classification: LCC RA448.5.A83 L44 2022 (print) | LCC RA448.5.A83
  (ebook) | DDC 362.1089/95073—dc23
LC record available at https://lccn.loc.gov/2021022985
LC ebook record available at https://lccn.loc.gov/2021022986

Printed in the United States of America

9 8 7 6 5 4 3 2 1

Contents

Acknowledgments

In the spring of 2009, my friend Michael emailed me to let me know that he was planning to complete his Clinical Pastoral Education (CPE) unit (the chaplaincy internship you'll read about in the Introduction) and wondered whether I'd planned to as well. I sighed. He and I had just completed a year of seminary coursework as part of our path to ordination in the Episcopal Church while we continued to hold full-time jobs. I had already let my colleagues at the University of California, Santa Barbara (UCSB), know that I was moving later that summer, so the thought of traveling every day to downtown Los Angeles to enter the hospital rooms of strangers left me preemptively exhausted. "It would be great if you could," Michael suggested in the last of our exchanges. Six weeks later, I joined Michael and four others—Mary Marjorie Bethea, David Erickson, Heather Erickson, and Norman Whitmire—in the "Cave," the conference room where, over the course of ten weeks during the summer of 2009, we listened to and held up each other as we muddled our way through stories of heartbreak, messiness, and, at times, joy. It was this experience of CPE, under the patient and wise direction of the Rev. Dr. Ronald David, that taught me to let stories breathe differently. This book might very well not exist if Michael hadn't nudged me. So thank you to the Rev. Michael Bell, who succeeded Ron at Good Sam Hospital as its chaplain, and to the others in my CPE unit.

I also give thanks to the two faith communities that have sustained me in my work as a priest: the people of St. Paul's Episcopal Church in Ventura, California, who sponsored my candidacy and the people of the Episcopal

Church of the Messiah in Santa Ana, California, whom I've had the honor of serving since 2012. I extend special gratitude to the Revs. Norma Guerra, Jerome Kahler, and Abel López; to the Rt. Revs. Diane Jardine Bruce, J. Jon Bruno, and John Taylor; and to Dr. David Sheridan. To my seminary colleagues and fellow priests in the Diocese of Los Angeles and beyond, I am grateful for this community of learning and faith: the Revs. Karri Backer, George Daisa, Greg Foraker, Nancy Frausto, Nicole Janelle, Bill Knutson, Julie Morris, and Anna Olson.

I joined the Department of Asian American Studies at the University of California, Irvine (UCI), after my CPE unit and count myself lucky to enjoy the company of colleagues and friends who are as generous as they are trenchant: Elaine Andres, Erica Cheung, Jennifer Choy, Robert Escalante, Dorothy Fujita-Rony, Laureen Hom, Claire Jean Kim, Julia Lee, Caroline McGuire, Annamarie Newton, Kasey Ning, Isa Quintana, Jasmine Robledo, Liz Clark Rubio, Ray San Diego, Beheroze Shroff, Linda Vo, and Judy Wu. Christine Balance moved away, but I cherished the many spontaneous conversations with my next-door officemate. Miss you, colleague! The wider constellation of colleagues at UCI has also nourished: Jonathan Alexander, Sharon Block, Philip Broadbent, Amy Chen, Youngmin Choe, Adrianne de Castro, Eleana Kim, Laura Kang, Rodrigo Lazo, Sei Lee, Stephen Lee, Julia Lupton, Glen Mimura, Sylvia Nam, Catherine Sameh, Jeanne Scheper, Jim Steintrager, Amanda Swain, and Tiffany Willoughby-Herard. I thank the Center for Medical Humanities staff for making concrete this important work at UCI—Sam Carter, JoAnn Jamora, and Makanani Salā—and the center's Executive Committee for its wise leadership: Adria Imada, Ketu Katrak, Jenny Terry, David Trend, and Drs. Tan Nguyen and Johanna Shapiro. I want to acknowledge and honor the center's founding director Douglas Haynes, who helped spearhead bringing medical humanities to UCI and for his continued support of this important endeavor. I thank Sarah Orem for her work in the Mellon Foundation Sawyer Seminar at UCI during the 2019–2020 academic year and for her fierce scholarship.

Chris Fan and Jerry Lee are also my UCI colleagues, but they are part of a special group of people who have been attending conferences hosted by the American Studies Association of Korea. These meetings have become indispensable for the critical exchange of ideas, meals, and *noraebang*. Other fellow travelers include Daniel Kim, Eun Joo Kim, Jinah Kim, Robert Ku, Heijin Lee, Anita Mannur, Kimberly McKee, and David Roh. I have also cherished the intellectual comradeship of colleagues in Korea, including Peggy Cho, the Very Rev. Nak-hyun Joseph Joo, Chang Hee Kim, the Rev. Ho-kwan Crispin Kim, Min-Jung Kim, Naomi Kim, Eunha Na, and Jae Roh. Special thanks to Kyung-Sook Boo for inviting me to give a talk at Sogang University based on an early draft of a chapter and to Hyungji Park for the many meals and conversations that were as sustaining as they were delicious. And to the *flâneur extraordinaire* of Seoul, Joe Jeon: here's to many more evenings of soju and dried squid while sitting on plastic chairs at 을지로 3가.

The Association for Asian American Studies (AAAS) represents the closest an academic organization can get to a spiritual home, and the reason it is for me and for so many others is that the AAAS, imperfectly, works to live into the intellectual imagination of a rigorous and shared—and sometimes contested— vision of social justice. Many I've already named are part of this association; here are a few more: Aimee Bahng, Crystal Baik, Leslie Bow, Jason Oliver Chang, Wendy Cheng, Floyd Cheung, Catherine Ceniza Choy, Lawrence-Minh Bùi Davis, Jigna Desai, Jennifer Kwon Dobbs, Lan Duong, Cat Fung, Theo Gonzalves, Jennifer Ho, Tammy Ho, Caroline Hong, Madeline Hsu, Betsy Huang, Jang Wook Huh, Jane Iwamura, Helen Jun, Miliann Kang, Grace Kim, Heidi Kim, Nadia Kim, Sue Kim, C. N. Le, Jeehyun Lim, Joo Ok Kim, Lili Kim, Daryl Maeda, Viet Thanh Nguyen, Crystal Parikh, Chris Perreira, Cathy Schlund-Vials, Sarita See, Nitasha Sharma, Min Hyoung Song, Oliver Wang, Ellen Wu, Karen Tei Yamashita, and Timothy Yu. I am deeply grateful to Patrick Anderson, Mel Chen, Lochlann Jain, Christine Lee, Lana Lin, Dr. Sunita Puri, and Brandy Worrall for engaging in person with me about their books. I hope that I was able to do justice to your work in mine.

Portions of this book were delivered at Boston College, Minzu University of China (Beijing), the Beijing Foreign Studies University, Sogang University, and UCSB. I thank my former colleagues in the Department of Asian American Studies for inviting me to do so: Diane Fujino, John Park, Lisa Park, and Xiaojian Zhao. (There is one more person in this department, but I'll save her for later.) I also was given the opportunity to present a portion of Chapter 2 as a keynote address at the Polish Association of American Studies (PAAS) in Warsaw in 2015 and, thanks to funding from the U.S. Embassy, presented papers at the University of Gdańsk, the Jagiellonian University, and the University of Warsaw during this extended trip. My thanks to Tomasz Basiuk, then the president of PAAS, for showing me such hospitality, and to Aneta Dybska, Dominika Ferens, and Zuza Ladya for their enduring friendship.

The group of graduate students who used to gather at our apartment to watch *The X-Files* in the 1990s has become a diaspora but continues to sustain me, despite the geographic distance: Anna Alves, Kelly Jeong, Mike Murashige, Minh Nguyen, Laura Pulido, Darlene Rodrigues, and Eric Wat. Same goes for the people at the University of California, Los Angeles, many of whom I have known longer as digital presences than analog but whose impact remains just as real: King-Kok Cheung, La'Tonya Rease Miles, and Richard Yarborough. I have also been fortunate to enjoy collegiality through the Yonsei International Summer School: Paul Chang, Peter Graham, Dan O'Neill, and Leslie Paik. I give thanks for SooJin and Sxela Pate, Joanna Brooks and David Kamper, and Ella and Rosa Brooks-Kamper for being wise and loving friends and interlocutors to me and my family.

I express my gratitude to Temple University Press and my editor, Shaun Vigil, whose enthusiasm and support for this project were unwavering and clearheaded. Thank you also to the press's staff for making this book an object in the world: Ann-Marie Anderson, Gary Kramer, Mary Rose Muccie, and Ashley Petrucci. Thank you to the series editors of *Dis/color* for their faith in my project: Nirmala Erevelles, Julie Avril Minich, and especially Cindy Wu for their guidance and constant support. I am grateful to the two readers of my manuscript who helped to make it much better; to Susan Deeks, the copyeditor who fixed my many mistakes; and to David Martinez for his work in developing the index. Thank you to Jean Shon for generously allowing me to have her photograph serve as the book's cover. The UCI Humanities Center provided funding for the index and the book cover photo; I am grateful for the support.

I want to name two people whose influence is everywhere in this book and in my intellectual life. I often say to my graduate students that there comes a point when a doctoral student knows more about their projects than their dissertation chairs. Mimi Khúc long ago passed that stage, but it gives me a special pride that she has become not only a colleague and dear friend, but someone I now consider my mentor. erin Khuê Ninh, the aforementioned unnamed faculty member of UCSB's Asian American Studies Department, and I shared drafts and meals and phone calls and text exchanges as we shaped our books, and it is not an overstatement to say that mine would not have been possible without her friendship, deep wisdom, and kindness. She is practically a coauthor; she is most definitely my North Star.

I thank my parents, John and Young Lee, for their support and for coming to California so they could have regular meals with their grandchildren, and to Jiyoun and Kun Ho Cho for their love from New Jersey. Love to my brother, Ted; my sister-in-law, Eun Kyoung; and my nephew, Hahnul. Mags, our then recently adopted rescue dog, was my writing companion for an entire year, and I am grateful for her non-anxious presence and for giving me a reason to take walks throughout the day when the writing stuck. And there is a special section in my heart that is a wellspring of love for which there is no limit: my children, Sona and Jihae, and my partner in life, Julie Cho. The book's done. Let's have dinner.

Pedagogies of Woundedness

Introduction

Sickness unto Death

An Asian American Learning

Model Minority Afterlives

"Hello, welcome," begins Julie Yip-Williams's memoir, *The Unwinding of the Miracle*, which chronicles her four-year journey with cancer, not to be overshadowed by her life as a disabled Vietnamese refugee. "This story begins at the ending. Which means that if you are here, then I am not," writes Yip-Williams.[1] By the time I would be able to read these words in February 2019, just as I was beginning this Introduction, she had been dead for almost a year. "But it's okay," Yip-Williams insists, a succinct, almost curt statement that seems to hold off one's gasp at reading the words of a ghost, an occult language. But surely the grief must be so tautly felt still, by her husband, their young daughters; this prologue completed just weeks before her death makes one almost not believe this insistence that her death is okay, that her forty-two-year life ends because of metastatic cancer. Still, she says it all the same, a rune through which she invites you and me to read her life story in which cancer is something that is—grudgingly? maddeningly?—okay. For it is cancer that kills her, but Yip-Williams won't utter the disease in this prologue. No, instead she reframes her memoir as one determined by her illness but not defined by it, or, as she puts it, "What began as a chronicle of an early and imminent death became—if I may be very presumptuous—something far more meaningful: an exhortation to you, the living."[2] As she unwinds in death, Yip-Williams gives, even presumes, herself to you and me, her readers, what Lauren Berlant will describe of her late friend Eve Kosofsky Sedgwick's scholarly work written during her cancer: "a training," a kind of learning, if you will. Yip-Williams exhorts us to "live while you're living, friends."[3] A simple enough epigraph, for sure, but knowing what we will know she will have gone through by the book's end, her imperative is a form of pedagogy that, her memoir demonstrates, can be learned only through the crucible of experience that is terminal illness.

Readers wanted to learn something from what she was teaching through her memoir. *The Unwinding of the Miracle* debuted in the top ten of the *New York Times* best-seller list in late February 2019.[4] The book is the final form of what began as a blog created by Yip-Williams when she received the diagnosis of stage IV colon cancer in 2013.[5] Among the many readers of her blog, *My Cancer Fighting Journey*, was Mark Warren, who would become her editor at Random House, the book's publisher. In the acknowledgments section, Yip-Williams's surviving family refers to Warren as a "friend," then thanks the "most important people to this enterprise: Julie's readers."[6] So popular was her blog that *CBS Sunday Morning* ran a story titled "Borrowed Time" featuring her and her family on March 11, 2018; eight days later, the *New York Times* published an obituary of Yip-Williams.[7] The presumption of a built-in audience for the book, and the outsize publicity that Yip-Williams received by the press shortly before and after her death, suggests that people sat at her digital bedside as she imparted her wisdom. In death, Yip-Williams's memoir would serve as her magnum opus that could teach a nation.

Why do people want to learn from someone like Julie Yip-Williams, and what is it that they want to learn? I mean: her death, tragic as it was, especially for her family, was one of more than 609,000 cancer-related deaths in 2018. Yip-Williams died at forty-two, five years after her diagnosis; her husband and two daughters survive her, a tragic milestone for the family to lose a partner and mother so young. But while uncommon, cancer among the young is not rare, and we will read stories of others even younger than she. Nor is her exhortation to the living "to live" an unfamiliar trope among those stricken with terminal illness. Both obituary and television profile accentuate Yip-Williams's admirable resilience in the face of her disease and the slow process of dying. "Truth is," the CBS reporter Tracy Smith says in her story, "Julie Yip-Williams has a sort of vision the rest of us might envy: the ability to see challenges, and even death, as opportunity, and to face them head-on and with gratitude."

I want to suggest that Yip-Williams's Asian American story determines the response she has received from her reading public. Her blog and book, as well as those who write about her and the book, all situate her cancer alongside the harrowed chronicle of her childhood: born in Vietnam into an ethnic Chinese family, baby Julie, her grandmother is horrified to discover, is blind; her grandmother orders her parents to find a way to kill her. Her parents' reluctance eventually turns into refusal, after which Julie and her family flee Vietnam and arrive in the United States, where surgery partially restores her sight (though she will remain legally blind). Her refugee parents toil away in nail salons and wholesale grocery; meanwhile, Julie attends Williams College and Harvard Law School and lands a position as an associate at a corporate law firm. She meets and marries Josh Williams, also a corporate lawyer who eventually makes partner at his firm; she gives birth to two girls. By all accounts, Yip-Williams's story is exemplar of the "success frame" that Asian Americans are supposed to have enjoyed in the past half century or so, a broad social narrative of educational and economic mobility that has captured the imaginations of social scientists who marvel at a racial group's meteoric rise and fuels the expectations and demands of Asian American (immigrant) parents who expect nothing less from their children.[8] The term that Asian Americanists have used to describe this narrative into which many Asian Americans fit, sometimes uneasily, sometimes enthusiastically—and, true, sometimes disavowed—is model minority discourse, a concept as banal and ubiquitous within Asian American formations and among Asian American studies scholars as it continues to be remarkable to those on the cultural and scholarly outside for whom the term still feels innovative.[9]

Nowhere in this classic model minority story that Yip-Williams seems to have enjoyed is there room for cancer and premature death. Yet cancer comes to her in 2013 and claims her five years later, leaving in her absence emotional devastation whose outpouring in part resulted in her memoir, a literary version of her afterlife. The memoir materializes a paradox that has haunted Asian Americans ever since the model minority became a social option—nay, an imperative—by which to live in the contemporary United States. Asian Americans must exemplify success, in the classroom and the workplace; by extension, they must also inhabit indefinitely healthy bodies that serve this success frame.[10] Yet they, too, get sick, become disabled, and, perhaps to the astonishment of their American readers, Asian Americans such as Julie Yip-Williams also die. The facticity of Asian American mortality seems absurd to write—I feel silly writing it—and yet the outpouring of affection for Yip-Williams and for her book suggests an un-ironic surprise that, indeed, model minority bodies not only can, but do, fail eventually, some sooner rather than later. This reality is simultaneously unbearable and unimaginable, *and* it must serve some kind of pedagogical enchantment, to fulfill in death what has been Asian America's role in life.[11]

Model Minority (Social) Science: "Grit"

All this seems so incredible and new, as if Asian Americans have started dying only recently, in large part because they've long been expected to be harbingers of nothing less than the good American life, showing the rest of the United States how it ought to be done.[12] Take, for instance, the latest iteration of model minority formation and figuration, this time crossing disciplines from sociology to psychology. Once the domain of Chicago School–inflected culturalist notions of success frame values as causation for Asian American achievement in, say, elite higher education and, later, adult income levels—from William Petersen in 1966 to Amy Chua in 2011—it now enters the neuropsychological domain in the noncognitive term "grit," popularized by the "MacArthur Genius" psychologist Angela Duckworth. In a TED talk in 2013 and book in 2016 she presents, through anecdote and more statistically "quantifiable" data, the idea that the ostensibly intangible affective quality of grit, defined loosely as "this combination of passion and perseverance that [makes] high achievers special," is the behavioral secret sauce to social and economic advancement, not innate talent or skill.[13] Notwithstanding the ways that her findings dovetail with prior studies that suggested that Asian American "grit" helped to explain their presence in U.S. elite universities, in contrast to the talent and leadership qualities of their white counterparts, the dimensions of grit are fashioned by Duckworth not to be confined to Asian Americans or to be solely biologically determined: parents or adults in households can (and should, in her mind) cultivate grit in their children by setting high expectation and direction to inculcate passion and perseverance for long-term goals.[14] Striking here, then, are the two bookend examples that emerge in Duckworth's book, both of them ensconcing grit within her own Asian American family: she concludes with a thought experiment of what her two daughters think of their mother's insistence on grit. "Amanda and Lucy wish I'd relax a little," Duckworth jokes, "and, you know, talk more about Taylor Swift. But they don't wish their mother was anything other than a paragon of grit."[15] The success frame affirmed in the next generation by the book's end provides neat closure to the book's opening, which contains, crucially and perhaps unwittingly, a narrative aporia.

In the book's prologue, Duckworth recounts the many times her father would say to her, "You're no genius," which she later interpreted as his determination to instill in her—through indefinitely deferred praise—the quality of grit that would define her career in psychology. Her receiving the MacArthur Fellowship and the subsequent book that houses this story of her seemingly emotionally fraught relationship with her father culminate at the prologue's end with a scene designed to bring to affective fruition the triumph of her insight as both rebuke *and* affirmation of her father's quip:

> When I finished writing [my book], I went to visit my dad. Chapter by chapter, over the course of days, I read him every line. *He's been battling Parkinson's disease for the last decade or so, and I'm not entirely sure how much he understood.* Still, he seemed to be listening intently, and when I was done, he looked at me. After what felt like an eternity, he nodded once. And then he smiled.[16]

This tableau is an Asian American daughter's fantasy: the taciturn but ultimately affirming immigrant parent who finally acknowledges his daughter's achievement, gives her in adulthood what he'd long denied in her younger years. It also offers a mirrored reversal of the parent-child dynamic, of the child now reading to her parent who is seemingly illiterate or otherwise incapable of reading himself. Indeed, Duckworth's recognition of her father's chronic illness, which in turn makes him and his bodily response to her recitation laconic to her observation, provides (at least) two divergent hermeneutical outcomes. On the one hand, because she can't fully "read" him in his wounded, ill body, Duckworth can't help but read his nod and smile as anything but parental assent to her grit *and* genius rather than, say, the acknowledgment that she'd just finished reading to him a very long book. And on the other hand, her affective demand to read to him even as she is either unable or unwilling to know what her father's body may be communicating through his illness—the possibility that her Parkinson-stricken father may develop desires beyond those attributable to grit, such as achievement and success and societal recognition—speaks to the profound limits of communicability when an Asian American daughter, formed in the pedagogy of the model minority, can't imagine a language beyond the ones that imagine both ultimate success and indefinite health via grit, her father's irrevocable disease notwithstanding.

That we ascribe an almost fairy tale-like expectation of Asian American life that is simply shocked at its possible finitude, let alone the inevitable end that is mortality—and the variety of ways that move Asian Americans toward their death—informs the question that is at the heart of this book. What happens when model minorities and their attachment, witting or not, to the narrative of progression confront the exigencies of illness and disability, the wounds of bodily failure? What different story, if any, might be possible? How do Asian Americans, intentionally and relentlessly cast to perform the codependent role of validating the American forms of (neo)liberalism, tell stories in light of the realism of illness that always—and here I must insist, *always*—puts the lie to the ableist fiction of indefinite health and able-bodiedness? What, indeed, is the learning from a book such as *Unwinding* that another such as Duckworth cannot quarter in theorizing Asian American "grit?" What happens when we aggregate illness as an Asian American condition and an emergent mode of narrative, collated and read together? And, conversely, what would be the consequences if Yip-Williams had not written the story of her illness as a constitutive part of her Asian American life? What might be the cost of not witnessing what happens when model minorities get sick and die?

Dying Offstage

Here's an example of the cost from my own experience as a teacher. On my teaching rota is an upper-division course titled "California in Asian American Fiction." The first two works that I assign are classics: Hisaye Yamamoto's collection of short stories and Kim Ronyoung's novel *Clay Walls*. I've taught both books for a very long time, so it surprised me that the last time I taught them I was struck by something that, until now, had seemed fairly marginal to their stories, in large part because they *are* marginal to the stories: men die in hospitals, alone. Here I'm thinking specifically of the Japanese immigrant and former internee Kasuyuki, or Charley, in "Las Vegas Charley" and the Korean immigrant Chun and second-generation Korean American Willie in *Clay Walls*.[17] All of them are stricken with some fatal disease: cirrhosis and cancer for Charley and tuberculosis for Chun and Willie. All three characters are not idealized masculine figures, even for the normative gender expectations of their day: Charley's addiction to both alcohol and gambling clearly index his tragic downward trajectory following the death of his wife, his incarceration during World War II, and his consignment to the most menial of jobs. Likewise, Chun's and Willie's attempts to mitigate their lower-class status in California through sexual violence—rape for Chun, sexual battery for Willie—make them, in Kim's narrative, the "wrong" guys for their respective partners, Haesu and Faye. Within the novel's ideological parameters, both men must die so that the women protagonists who occupy higher classes can eventually partner with men of a similar social status: Min, the poet scholar, joins Haesu's household, and Faye receives a letter from Daniel, which portends the beginning of a demonstrably middle-class (model minority?) second generation.

But I found myself following the men left to die alone, offstage. I wanted to follow them not because I find them sympathetic at all, or to understand—

and certainly not to excuse—their moral failings. I wanted to follow them because these are men whose ends we are not allowed to see, their physical anguish witnessed by no one, whose suffering may be beyond the horizons of imagination of their creator. What does it mean for an author to cite and not pursue characters who suffer intensely? What does it mean for a writer to leave her character behind? What does that unimagined suffering look like, and what analytical, methodological, and theoretical resources are necessary to marshal to attend to that suffering?

These men's actions can't be redeemed. Particularly for Chun, his raping of Haesu demands an accounting, for sure. But just as Chun's sexual violence is not justified, the novel's resolution to the contradiction that Haesu (and Faye) must overcome to pursue a model minority dream just beginning to take shape in the post–World War II household they inhabit by the novel's end is unjust. Not allowing Kim's and Yamamoto's unsympathetic men to die alone might give us a means to theorize what it might mean to refuse to let the suffering of another, however despicable, go unimagined. To refuse to cross the threshold to enter the spaces of men left to die and suffer alone is connected to a general refusal to let Asian Americans be anything other than model minorities who must, in our imaginations, therefore live forever. The guys who die? Let them die alone, forgotten.

At some point, though, you have to acknowledge the body in the other room. So you cross the threshold and wonder what meaning to take from what you witness. So many people followed Yip-Williams's journey through her cancer and stayed by her side as she died, by way of her blog; so many more have witnessed her end by reading her posthumous memoir. Model minorities, those on whom we have projected every fantasy of unlimited social mobility and progress, will surely die, their bodies failing them despite their, and our, well-intentioned wishes. So surely there must be something to learn from them, from her. Answering *this* question is especially important for those of us invested in a deep critique of the very formation of the model minority—those of us in, say, Asian American studies whose political and ideological commitments lie in the demolition of such a dangerous identity formation that has been mobilized to batter other people of color and straitjacket Asian Americans into forms of social and economic collusion that are, in the final instance, toxic to themselves. Like capitalism's waste degrading the planet, the surpluses of investing in the model minority, Asian American studies insists, are the invisible wounds of contemporary debt peonage that manifest in, at best, emotional trauma and, all too often, suicide—what we should more accurately call self-murder. For Asian Americans, it is the specter of the model minority's vanishing that does the killing. Those of us committed to ending the tyranny of the model minority in Asian American life work to imagine a capacious social formation, toward a heretofore untrodden terrain of interaction in which the complications of life—indeed, the very ideas of complex personhood—are reimagined and restored to those otherwise consigned to bare life, Asian American and beyond.

This has been, of course, the political project of Asian American studies. But I would suggest that our field has long been unable to think, and therefore live, Asian American embodiment beyond the model minority because such an alternative remains premised on a futurity and imagination of a body that is healthy, not ill. Activism is chiefly imagined as an activity by an able-bodied person who can move autonomously in time and space; it is still hard to imagine doing something recognized as political while lying in bed. (I will, however, imagine the supine position as a bodily form of activism in the Epilogue.) There's a certain cruel logic to this, given how historically the intersection of disability and racial/gender identities have mutually reinforced social denigration of people who are not white men.[18] It's still hard to set aside the ableist logic if your life depends on it.[19] Asian American studies also, and still, does not imagine its central subject as one, say, consigned to a hospital bed as its imagined or inevitable or desirable future. To this extent, this image—and the inevitability that this image represents, that we will (yes, even model minorities and those who disavow that ideological hailing) get ill, die—remains another world, another species, beyond imagination, *even though this ill body is our future.*

In between disavowal and inevitability lies a different way of interpreting and living in the world. For those whose bodies and minds are not normatively celebrated present an alternative ethos summed up in a question Tobin Siebers asked his whole life: "What would it mean to esteem the disabled [and ill] body for what it really is?"[20] And what this body really is is okay, on its own, in its own terms, notwithstanding biomedicine's desire to find in it deficit, pathology, and deformity, a body in need of treatment. The ideologies and violence of cure, of a body that can be restored "back" to an idealized nondisabled state of being, are what make disabled lives miserable, disability studies teaches, not the bodies in and of themselves.[21] A version of Asian American studies that it might tell, then, is a story with which disability studies could resonate: as a field of study and life practice that tells stories about how differently marked bodies have made a difference in the fetch of their lives. Asian American studies insists that, to know with some fidelity the truth of our differently marked bodies, it is necessary to learn the narratives that have overdetermined them—history, discourse, ideology, policy—and listen to what these marked bodies say: anger, resignation, protest, suicide, assimilation. This version may come alongside disability studies, look at the Asian American body marked as different and esteem it for what it is. Yet in an attempt to account for the damage done, the field continues its slippage on finding a form of cure, from the model minority's curative violence toward a fantasy of an a priori state of being not already differentially marked. But the pursuit of justice calls for a tenderness toward our wounds, not their cosmetic removal.

This disavowal explains in large part why a memoir such as Yip-Williams's has been available for readers only in the very recent past, why Asian Americans have been late in writing about becoming ill, deciding that the experience of woundedness born of illness or disability was worth telling. The "memoir boom" that many have noted marks the contemporary moment, G. Thomas Couser suggests, is crucially linked to a "boom in disability [and by extension, illness] writing," which he considers "the most important development in American life writing in the last three decades or so and thus a cultural and historical phenomenon of great significance."[22] The rise of the illness memoir signals a dramatic shift toward taking seriously the need and desire not only to write about diseased and disabled bodies, but, indeed, to take seriously the strange idea that ill and disabled bodies might *desire*, and that this desire need not be only the desire to be healthy and not disabled. The genre itself then becomes a platform to persuade readers that there may be something unimaginably desirable in reading a story of illness beyond one that simply results in recovery, one that cultivates a new ethos valued for what it is: the ill narrator's uptake.[23] Correspondingly, the emergence of disability studies within both the social sciences and humanities that, among many things, calls chiefly to undo the ideology of ability, as Tobin Siebers puts it—and, perhaps in a more porous way, the work in illness studies and medical/health humanities by scholars such as Arthur Frank and Rita Charon—diversely points toward a scholarly capacity that at once critiques the cultural obsession with health and able-bodiedness and provides routes to empathy, justice, and care for the bodies from which stories and illness emerge.[24] We might call this "boom" a movement of sorts whose rallying cry goes something like this: you will get ill, your body will crumble, and you will die, and that is all right. Once Asian Americans simply had to wander off into the wilderness to die alone, save for maybe a lonely family member. It's taken us a long time to wonder whether there is value in following them on this final journey.

To move indelibly away from able-bodied as both ideal and normative thus helps us understand what, until very recently, was the relative dearth of illness stories written by Asian Americans amid at the sea of stories that

Couser cites and about which he writes.[25] This is not to say that there *should* be proportionally as many Asian American narratives about illness and disability; rather, it is to note that there aren't that many and to ask why. In writing about her polio-borne disability, the Asian American studies scholar Sucheng Chan suggests that the silence among Asian American households regarding an ill or disabled loved one stems from a belief that, in "East Asian cultures, there is a strong folk belief that a person's physical state in this life is a reflection of how morally or sinful he or she lived in previous lives."[26] She extends this idea of collective, transgenerational culpability into viewing bodies no longer fully able or healthy as cultural tendency toward verbal ridicule or the shame of silence. This notion that Chan advances doesn't originate from her, and I will insist that it doesn't actually originate from Asian American communities. Where this notion of Asian and Asian American aversion to illness and disability comes from is the reproduction both in popular culture and scholarly language that reinforces this discourse as indigenous to Asian American communities. "Asian families," writes Irmo Marini in the most recent edition of *The Psychological and Social Impact of Illness and Disability* (2012), "tend to be secretive of family problems and often do not want to divulge the family shame."[27] Given the authoritative stamp of approval by medical, psychological, and other cultural brokers, this discourse of shame that explains the silence of Asian Americans toward their experience of woundedness thus provides a culturalist rationale to Asian American reticence to writing stories about their disabled and ill bodies: they are ashamed of the forms of embodiment that aren't normatively healthy and able.

But if there is a kernel of truth to this disavowing of the ill and disabled body within Asian America, then what fuels this desire toward health is the parallel captive imagination that Asian Americans wield in relation to that other mode of social "perfection": the model minority, of which Yip-Williams was a member, at least until cancer stripped her of this social citizenship. erin Khuê Ninh insists that the model minority is not only a "myth" imposed by white society to discipline Asian Americans into compliant subjects to the U.S. nation-state and capitalist logic, but *also* a discourse internalized by Asian American communities and families as values around which to mobilize: "The assimilationist, individualist, upwardly mobile professional class of the model minority *is*, for familial intents and purposes, Asian America's model children."[28] It is the model minority that insists that Asian America's children enjoy the bodies that make their upward mobility not only possible but necessary in an economic system built on ableism and health as its paragon. And this possessive investment in normatively desirable bodies means not simply the maintenance of the presumably healthy body you're born with, but also its constant cultivation, a neurotic care of the self that can optimize one's economic potential, one's human valuation.[29] What is really at stake is the extent to which the ideology of able-bodiedness typifies the allegiance to racial and gender ideologies of an ideal *Asian American* body, dancing—for many happily, for others miserably—in the larger constellation of the reproduction, medicalization, and industrialization of the *healthy* and nondisabled model minority.

Physician Authors: The Tragic Heroes of Asian America

Nowhere is this impulse to inhabit and narrate the self in ableist, model minority relation to illness, disability, and woundedness more prevalent than in the narratives of those called to care for wounded bodies: Asian American medical and other health-care practitioners. Indeed, prior to the most recent emergence of illness narratives, the "boom" in memoirs by Asian Americans were written largely from the vantage of physicians. And why not? According to the Association of American Medical Colleges, almost one in four students in U.S. medical schools is of Asian descent, a ratio that vastly outstrips the proportion of Asian Americans in the general U.S. population (though not a number that is an outlier if considered next to enrollment in elite undergraduate colleges and universities, where Asian Americans also experience disproportionate overrepresentation).[30] And on the surface, what genre of life writing better affirms the model minority trajectory than that of the young Asian American who toils away in dissection, pores through anatomy and physiology books, memorizes pathologies and diagnoses ad nauseam, deprives herself of sleep and pleasure during internship and residency, and sacrifices a sexual and social life for the sake of her vocation? What mode of identity is better suited to putting forth the notion that Asian American bodies do not fall ill but, instead, are the paragons of making ill and disabled bodies better, the socially perfect lifting up of the socially wounded? Certainly, this model minority medical narrative template has given young Asian American doctors a public platform: Michelle Au's *This Won't Hurt a Bit* (2011) and Anthony Youn's *In Stitches* (2011) humorously depict the travails and anxieties of enduring medical school while also negotiating the tricky dimensions of culture, race, and gender and sexual politics within and outside the classroom and hospital. As Au writes toward the end of her memoir, on the brink of winning an anesthesiology fellowship: "We continue to work hard, amplify our experience and confidence, and hope that soon enough, our self-image will catch up to the outward image that we project."[31] Both, however, retain the impulse to not relate their own bodies to the broken ones they encounter and treat, and for the many people they encounter, both Au's and Youn's subjectivities remain resolutely monadic in relation to illness: their patients get sick, but they do not.

Within this faith in the primacy of the Asian American model minority physician whose health and capacity to cure makes him an idealized narrative form for contemporary U.S. readers, physician authors of South Asian descent enjoy special reputations as the paragons of medical pedagogy. As members of a large cohort of immigrant doctors that came from the Subcontinent after the general passage of the 1965 Immigration and Nationality Act, which included specific provisions to coax what were then called "foreign medical graduates" (FMGs) to relieve the United States of its health-care staffing shortage, South Asian Americans have constituted the largest group of immigrant physicians in the United States, with the American Association of Physicians of Indian Origin (AAPI) claiming membership of more than fifty thousand.[32] The presence of South Asian American physicians has been ubiquitous in the United States for more than a half-century; it's not uncommon to find these brown men (and women, but mostly men) in places that white doctors have largely abandoned, such as rural communities or urban spaces of intense and chronic poverty. Of Asian Americans in U.S. medical schools, South Asians consistently constitute the largest demographic when the data are disaggregated.[33] So it's perhaps not surprising that the *narrative* authority that they wield seems to have come suddenly, almost surreptitiously. It is clear that today the public face of U.S. medicine is decidedly South Asian. Atul Gawande, general surgeon at Brigham and Women's Hospital in Boston, is also a *New Yorker* contributor and the author of four books, the latest of which, *Being Mortal*, was on the *New York Times* best-seller list for twenty-seven weeks; a Public Broadcasting System (PBS) documentary by the same title was produced in 2015, with Gawande as principal narrator.[34] Jeff Bezos of Amazon, Warren Buffet of Berkshire Hathaway, and Jamie Dimon of JP Morgan Chase tapped Gawande to head up Haven, a new health-care company created ostensibly to fix the endemically broken health-care cost and delivery system (he left when the COVID-19 pandemic broke out).[35] *The Emperor of All Maladies* (2010), Siddhartha Mukherjee's biography of cancer, was named by *Time* magazine as one of the top one hundred books of the past century, and PBS recently broadcast a three-part, six-hour version by the same title, produced by Ken Burns, with Mukherjee as main medical consultant.[36] Mukherjee's latest book, *The Gene: An Intimate History*, also enjoyed best-seller status.[37] Abraham Verghese, an infectious disease specialist at Stanford University, has written three best-selling books, including a novel; his TED talk in 2011, "A Doctor's Touch," has enjoyed more than one million views; and in 2015 President Barack Obama selected Verghese to be a recipient of the National Humanities Medal.[38] Obama's last Surgeon General of the United States was Vivek Murthy, then a thirty-eight-year-old internist educated at Harvard and Yale.[39] In 2016, Paul Kalanithi wrote (and his wife completed) the poignant memoir *When Breath Becomes Air* about his life as a rising neurosurgeon and his sudden diagnosis of a brain malignancy; when Kalanithi died, his book was also a *New York Times* best seller.[40] That same year, another book by a South Asian American physician captured attention: Prabhjot Singh's *Dying and Living in the Neighborhood*, a reflection on health care at the "street level" based on his work serving a community in New York's Harlem neighborhood.[41]

This tableau that I offer, of South Asian American (male) physicians and surgeons hailed not only as exceptional doctors but also as narrators and leaders of contemporary U.S. medicine, begs at least two questions, which I try to answer in Chapter 1 of this book: what does it mean that the face of modern medicine is a brown Asian man and that the person telling a very important, perhaps hegemonic, story of medicine is South Asian? What does it mean that South Asian American men are currently those most trusted with questions about health care; about the experience of illness; about healing, suffering, and mortality? Through memoir and essay these physicians deliver resonant prose that attends to and mitigates the crisis in the biopolitical management of contemporary medicine. Readers may barely notice their brownness, as the authors themselves rarely cite their racial difference from their putative readers. This matters little, as their professional and institutional credentials themselves serve as amply expressive markers of their model minority embodiment and their appeal to white readerly desire—a virtuoso signaling.[42] As South Asian American practitioners and authors, they have been cast as health-care gurus, with all of the Orientalist yogi baggage attached to this term; as model minority exemplars to guide their readers, their present and future patients, to imagining ailing, ill, and suffering bodies as somehow all right. South Asian American physicians have made their medical excellence its own racial form.

But this making all right of illness, and even death, militates against medical ontology; contemporary biomedicine's ethos remains the extension of biological life even as, phenomenologically, such "life" appears less and less human. As organs fail in human bodies, physicians and other health-care professionals resort to and rely on medical technology as prosthetics and proxies, a giving over to a paradoxical fiction: doctors can keep their patients alive perhaps indefinitely if these people-turned-patients submit themselves fully to a medical regime that turns their bodies into terrains on which medical machines function as a form of "life." Jeffrey Bishop, a moral philosopher and physician himself, puts the conundrum this way: "Dead anatomy begets physiology; physiology begets technology; technology—the replacing of a dead organ by a dead machine—begets a life worse than death."[43] The reduction to little more than a form of bare life that characterizes the latter days of medical care thus explains the desperate need for something amounting to beauty or eloquence—or, at the very least, poignancy—that these South Asian American physician writers exhibit in their prose. Their words serve as proxies to forms of healing that biomedical procedure and technology cannot, these men marrying the scientific authority of model minority physicians with the postcolonial salve of South Asian literary cultural erudition. The man of science and the man of art are brought together once again in a warm-blooded physician writer who was rent asunder by the very scientific revolutions that propelled medicine to its ostensibly salvific status by making its practitioners cruelly cold to those they were saving. It is no surprise, then, that Gawande's *Being Mortal*, covered in Chapter 1, won him such acclaim, for who better than a South Asian American doctor, an attending surgeon at one of the most prestigious hospitals in the United States (Brigham and Women's Hospital), to teach people how to die well and as meaningfully as Asian American model minorities ostensibly have taught their American colleagues how to live well?

Indeed, the perforce challenge for Asian American physicians is to be deeply formed in the image of the model minority and all of its attendant social rewards of status, resources, and general affirmation and to turn this into a pedagogy that pivots away from medical fantasy and toward a clinical realism in which patients—and physicians—get sick and die. What in *this* story, in these scenes that are the only elements that are inevitable in the contingencies of illness and health care, are model minority physicians to do? As they witness their patients take the inexorable turn toward death, physicians opt generally for one of two modalities. The first is to lean into their training and perform action without ceasing, to fine-tune diagnostic and treatment algorithms, to engage in what are called "heroic measures." This is the physician whose tireless advocacy for patients gets him coverage in the news, the doctor who manages to save all but the rare and unlucky few on television series about hospital medicine. This is the physician the rigors of medical education and residency are designed to produce, the building up of endurance after this many consecutively unslept hours to develop the stamina to do all in the service of keeping people alive, night and day. This is also the physician willing to subject his patients to every form of machinery needed to keep vital signs going, narcotizing them to the point of unconsciousness to prevent them from pulling on tubes and wires and stop the suffering born of the devices keeping them alive, a curative violence.[44]

At a certain point, however, medical heroism gives way to the denouement of embodied realism, the inevitability of death, which counts normatively in medicine as failure. In Chapter 2, each of our model minority physicians must confront the fact that sickness unto death is as inexorable and ubiquitous as those they are able to keep alive over the course of their careers as doctors. Asian American physician authors such as Michelle Au and Audrey Young employ different affective registers to mediate this reality—Au uses absurdist humor; Young, self-righteous idealism—and strive to hold at bay the foreboding. But patient deaths inevitably arise in their emergent careers, first as students, later as residents, and they are at a loss for words, their humor and their idealism lost in the chaos of confusion over vocational crisis. How to live with the realization that no amount of incremental or tectonic progress in medical science can obviate the body's eventual, and sometimes sudden, decline? Physicians who confront this question reckon, then, with a second modality to mortal realism. For a surgeon such as Pauline Chen, whose memoir engages this very question of reckoning with the mortality of her patients, one answer is to pivot away from the active pursuit of "fixing" ailing, broken bodies toward a capacious pause, an opening that allows patients' illness and dying to become something to behold as a stage of life that must be honored rather than simply medical failure. Chen calls this the vocation of the physician as healer, one who attends to people in illness and death not to eradicate disease but to bear witness to their ends. In short, Chen's story is one of a doctor turned chaplain, one tasked with reenchanting the clinical space of the hospital room into a contemporary form of *Ars moriendi*, a vocation no longer to prevent death but to find a way, within the bounds of her Hippocratic oath, to welcome it.

Gawande and Chen thus close their chapters on Asian American medical memoir with an unresolved contradiction between structure and intention. On the one hand, both take the logic of medical heroism to its very end and find in its unrelenting infliction of suffering in the name of medical soteriology neither salvation nor solace but, instead, the profanity of meaningless bodily injury to the ill, dying person. Both wish to wrest from medicine's death drive that ironically demands clinical (bare) life not simply a modicum of compassion but a full-throated restoration of agency to people for whom such liberal identity was taken away when they became patients. This is what Chen hopes for when she imagines her attending and attention to the dying as the practice of a "healer" (as opposed to one who cures), a giving back of personhood to someone's last moments of life. For both Gawande and Chen, such a pivot requires a form of medical passivity, a deliberate recalibration of medical algorithm in which nonaction and nonapplication of medical expertise is the highest form of care. And yet only the most accomplished and skilled physician can craft withdrawal as good medical care rather than malpractice; only a physician gifted also as a wordsmith can turn what might otherwise look like shoddy diagnostic observation into narrative scenes of pathos and sentimentality, to revel in poetry rather than scientific language as linguistic balm. In a word, only model minority physicians are granted the authority to let go of their patients as an act of medical love rather than heartlessness, the ones able to frame the deaths of their patients as stories of success, even if full of inevitable grief.

But letting go is not the same as giving up, and it is this latter intention—giving up—that can never be an option for physicians. Model minorities and doctors they must remain, as inclined toward chaplaincy as they may be, lest they give themselves over to a wholly different form of care outside biomedical surveillance and attendant biopolitical management. So the contradictions endure: we want our physicians to be present at our end, to witness our deaths and mitigate our suffering, *and* because doctors such as Chen and Gawande commit to staying in the room, they remained tethered to hierarchies of medical structures and authority. They still write our death notes; they still tell our bodies' stories on the medical charts. They watch us die with all the care and empathy they can muster *and*, in the end, we are gone and medical futurity is ensured. Our deaths may move Asian American physicians, even transform them to take better care of future patients. But physicians' memoirs remain captive to an imagination where doctors remain the principal agents, perhaps even all the more so if they are recognized for forms of care beyond what has become expected in contemporary industrialized health care.

Asian American Illness Memoirs: What the Body Tells

This is why, late as their arrival has been, the emergence of Asian American illness memoirs in this contemporary moment constitutes among the most important—and possibly most treacherous—cultural developments in recent U.S. history. For illness narratives, stories told by people with and about their illnesses, stories told through their ill, wounded bodies, can represent—as *no physician's memoir can*—just how disruptive and transformative illness is to the person who experiences it. Illness most immediately and viscerally wrecks a person's self story and leaves in its wake and realization what Ronald Dworkin calls narrative wreckage. "The illness story is wrecked," writes the medical sociologist Arthur Frank, "because its present is not what the past was supposed to lead up to, and the future is scarcely thinkable."[45] All the more so for Asian Americans formed in the image of the success frame, for whom past activities serve as necessary and often painful investments for better, richer, and presumably healthier futures. (This explains in large part why medical ambitions are model minority hopes par excellence, for what profession promises more economic and social payoffs after a particularly grueling period of training and self-sacrifice than the movement from medical student/resident to attending physician?) Illness dashes the expectations of past performance securing the better present, and chronic or terminal illnesses auger the destruction of the fantasy and futurity of restoration or restitution as an option. Illness plunges our model minorities into indelible crisis and chaos.

Take, for instance, a sick Asian American deeply critical of model minority formation even when he was bodily healthy. Almost three years after receiving a diagnosis of colon cancer in the summer of 2006, the radical activist and artist Fred Ho composed his most "difficult to write" diary entry in the winter of 2009. Despite the optimistic prognosis of his doctors that a new tumor was not a relapse of previous tumors removed and blasted by chemotherapy, Ho refuses this medical narrative of progress and instead writes that he has reached a nadir in his experience of illness: "For the first time in this brutal cancer war, I was trapped in a vortex of depression, feeling I could not win, that I was getting worse, unable to do anything. . . . I began to feel suicidal—that giving up and dying would be preferable to living at a minimal existence."[46] With this, Ho signals his break from the normative notions of contemporary embodiment that demand health and wellness as the ideal to which all are expected to assent, so that even if someone does fall ill on occasion, the expectation is for that body to regain health at some future, inevitable time. But trying to imagine a future in which the body never regains "health" is so unimaginable that it leads Ho, otherwise and in the past full of vibrancy and vitality, down this emotional road of despair in which death is preferable to the "minimal existence" of ill embodiment. It is at this point that the totality of his cancer's disruptive power bears down on Ho, demolishing the remnants of a past self in which his illness was not a primary definer. He is reduced to "doing nothing," which makes of his life one worse than death. Ho is, in this moment, a wreck.

This moment of crisis, this break from the narrative of restitution and medical rescue, inaugurates for the first time, and perhaps unwittingly, in Ho's memoir, *Diary of a Radical Cancer Warrior: Fighting Cancer and Capitalism at the Cellular Level* (2011), an alternative identity and agency not hitched to his prior allegiance to health and the medical discourse that attempts to render all but the healthy, nondisabled body as desirable. It's an opening that he will, here and throughout his memoir, ultimately disavow and refuse: after this low point, as we will see in Chapter 3, Ho will recommit to an able and healthy body as the only desirable one, this time based on naturopathic treatment rather than allopathic medicine. But Ho's descent into chaos opens him and his readers to a psychic imagination and agency that, if pursued, might begin to cohere around something qualitatively different from one's submission to the medical regime. "The truth of the chaotic body," Arthur Frank writes, "is to reveal the hubris of other stories. Chaos stories show how quickly the props that other stories depend on can be kicked away."[47] These "other stories" are principally the restitution stories—I was once healthy, then I got sick, but I'll get better again—to which medicine insists we yoke our destinies, at almost all costs, until what constitutes "life" is composed of machines performing the work that failing organs cannot. Ho's narration of feeling "trapped," ironically, gestures to a form of freedom from hegemony of expectation that the fully restored body be a social compulsion. His commitment to health makes his illness unlivable, so he must either imagine a different narrative for himself to live differently or, under the demands of ableism, he must die.

It's a question that the other memoirists in Chapter 3 will broach, to different effect and affect from Ho's. Chapter 3 also takes up Brandy Liên Worrall's memoir *What Doesn't Kill Us* (2014), self-published because, as she shared with me in private correspondence, editors told her that "yet another cancer" memoir wouldn't be of interest to readers.[48] That, of course, was un-true, given both the increasing readership in publications about illness and, in particular, cancer stories *and* the trade houses' insatiable desire to put as many of these into print. It *is* possible that in 2014 editors weren't interested in an *Asian American* cancer or illness narrative, thanks to short-sighted un-derstandings of affective identification with an ill narrator who isn't white for a presumably white reader. As Keith Wailoo has suggested, the whiteness of cancer has held for a very long time: the entry, empowerment, and individu-alization of white women into early twentieth-century modernity made them biologically prone to cancer, whereas the degradations of exploitation, harsh labor, and poverty relegated nonwhites to premature death by other means. "Early-twentieth century public discourse," Wailoo writes, "placed not only womanhood but also privileged, civilized whiteness at the core of emerging cancer awareness."[49] This consciousness raising took the form of "communi-cating with vulnerable white women, using novels, magazines, films, mass media, and doctor-patient encounters to stress feminine vulnerabilities," the long-term aggregate effect of which is the cultivation and reproduction of the very readership that, trade publishers believe, want to read stories about women like them.[50] Asian Americans, of course, have required exceptional capacity and, as somatic corollary, honed, disciplined, and healthy bodies as prophylactic to vulnerabilities and risk, which explains why Worrall's rendition of the cancer story spends as much, if not more, time unpeeling the toxicities born of her failure to thrive in the success frame demanded of her Vietnamese refugee mother (and her post-traumatic stress disorder-plagued, drug- and alcohol-addicted Vietnam veteran white father) than of the horrors of being diagnosed and treated for breast cancer at thirty-one. At turns resolute and undone, grateful and resentful, Worrall presents a complicated and contradictory narrative persona through her illness, which she then connects recursively to an intergenerational and intersubjective story of collective, familial wounding: her cancer is not just analogous to her mother's "craziness" and her father's psychic and somatic maladies. Rather, her breast cancer is a material manifestation of the war in Vietnam that brought her parents together and devastated (at least) two communities: a Vietnamese one flung into diaspora and one traumatically sent back home only to fester, a ravaged land and body. Her cancer is the war's afterlife.

This was still (to remind) 2014, so publishers didn't think readers had much to learn from Worrall's story, to their editorial discredit. But within a year a story would emerge that cemented Asian American illness as offering something critical and crucial that made for necessary reading: Paul Kalanithi, a Stanford-trained neurosurgeon and child of Indian immigrants, was beginning to write and interview about how stage IV lung cancer interrupted his meteoric medical rise in neurosurgery. This captivated readers: an Asian American doctor who, by all accounts, should have lived the life a model minority is supposed to live now telling a story of illness that demolished this success narrative, as terminal illness is wont to do. No amount of cultural formation developed from his South Asian upbringing, at once both commonplace and liberal—his parents don't force him to study medicine—is sufficient ballast to protect Kalanithi from the contingency of illness. So a kind of sentimental affect must be forged, similar to that of Yip-Williams's memoir, to make the tragedy of Kalanithi's eventual death shot full of meaning, meaning worth learning.

But what do we learn in reading Kalanithi's memoir, *When Breath Becomes Air* (2016)? What do model minorities whose lives feel as if they end prematurely teach their readers, who seem suddenly to have needed this narrative pedagogy? The potential for these memoirs is also its possible treachery. For as much as writing a story of illness and the prospect of one's death might create narrative and affective space to imagine life no longer as a model minority, it can just as well work to join readers with the author's sentimental desire to take pleasure, even if grief-filled pleasure, in the short Asian American life as a good one, worth feeling at the expense of examining. This is, of course, exactly what Lauren Berlant identified as the primary affective engine of the sentimental, to curate what she calls an "intimate public" born of these shared feelings. "The turn to sentimental rhetoric," Berlant writes, "at moments of social anxiety constitutes a generic wish for an unconflicted world, one wherein structural inequities, not emotions and intimacies, are epiphenomenal. In this imaginary world the sentimental subject is connected to others who share the same sense that the world is out of joint, without necessarily having the same view of the reasons or solutions: historically, the sentimental intervention has tended to involve mobilizing a fantasy scene of collective desire, instruction, and identification that endures within the contingencies of the everyday."[51] Read, then, the story of a once-thriving Asian American who got sick and died to maintain the fantasy that the life of success is worth living all the same, shortened as it might be: it is *still* a *good* life. Its ethical legitimacy reinforced, the model minority thrives in its afterlife as readers imbue it simultaneously with the desire for this unconflicted world of indefinite health and the solidarity of securing this good life, no longer available to the now dead author, to those who now benefit from their story. Beneficiaries include readers for certain, these students of their deceased teachers of the only good life worth living. But they also include the author's actual children: both Yip-Williams's and Kalanithi's memoirs end with classic deathbed scenes reminiscent of their Victorian predecessors, once commonplace but increasingly rare because of the preponderance of clinical deaths in hospitals over the course of the twentieth century. As they lie dying, they are flanked by partners, parents, other familial loved ones, and their children, as if to highlight in this signal moment of loss the countervailing sentiment of hope that derives from the material futurity in the bodies of the authors' respective children.

The potentiality and potential treachery of the Asian American illness memoir must straddle an ethical incommensurability whose haunting is constitutive of its production. Born of the body's betrayal from the demand that it be healthy and able-bodied, the Asian American fallen ill writes a differential story of her embodiment, a narrative no longer tethered to the fantasy of restitution. Christine Lee's memoir, *Tell Me Everything You Don't Remember* (2016), chronicles the aftermath of her stroke at thirty-three, as well as the life she lived before this signal bodily crisis. Imagining this different relationship to a body now wounded by catastrophe invites her to reflect on the ways that insisting on a disciplined, healthy body that mirrors the socially and economic productive life she is expected to live as a model minority reveals the deeply toxic dimensions of such a life.[52] The congenital "hole in [her] heart" that allows the blood clot to pass on to her brain that engenders the stroke becomes a metaphor for how her model minority life, which begins with her debt-boundedness toward her parents and is later reinforced by her marriage to her white, tech-inclined husband, allows a variety of affective coping mechanisms—emotional invulnerability, attachment to mental fortitude, disavowal of bodily pain—is both source and symptom of an unsustainable way of living that will crumble after the stroke's occurrence. "My life fell apart," Lee writes in her memoir, "and then it rebuilt. Everything healed. And life started again."[53] But this "healing" reorients Lee toward a different relationship to her body based on attention, not disavowal; toward a different relationship to relations based on earnest intimacy, not acerbic wit; and toward a different relationship with her Asian American origins based on reckoning with her parents' historical connection to warfare, displacement, and trauma rather than reliving this connection. Lee calls this a "new resilience" that allows her no longer to be at war with her body, which is what allowed her to ignore the signs of the impending shock of the stroke.

But it is precisely this "new resilience" that runs the risk of sliding back into marshaling the wounded body for productive purposes, the Asian American ill body reenlisted into the broader contemporary project to demand of all bodies—able, disabled, ill—something worth learning, the memoir as index of neoliberalism's logic of value extraction from even the disaster of individual illness. This pedagogy of memoir as a demand to figure out "resilience" in the face of woundedness, to develop more capacities of "healing" to "start again," requires of Asian Americans such as Lee a didactic role in sickness that prolongs the productive capacities even into ill, disabled, and wounded experience. The threat of illness stories best exemplified by former model minorities waylaid by their broken bodies, yet no longer exempted from the imperatives of productivity, comes in the form of a narrative of affective recuperation. In coming to terms with this differently-abled body, Lee proffers a desire that shows, and thus reinforces rather than challenges, the very logic of value that pushed someone like her toward bodily collapse. The model minority is a haunt that is awfully hard to exorcise.

Illness and the Scholarly Monograph as Witness: Theirs and Mine

The specter of Michel Foucault is never far away, either. As much as we may want to provide those who have suffered through their travails of illness and medical treatment, to tend to their wounds by their bedsides, we can't help but wonder whether our very attachment to an Asian American story of illness isn't yet another iteration of a deeper logical impulse to channel every story, even stories of "failure" such as a chronic or terminal illness, to serve and advance the discourse of human capital optimization. Can we find a self within or beyond discursive capture? Who better to ask than those whose professional lives require them to think through "critical theory" *and* who themselves have felt the viscerality and vulnerabilities of bodies undone by illness and disability—that is, academic scholars whose intellectual formations are both interrupted and informed by bodily woundedness by way of disease and other forms of toxicity? Chapter 4 introduces three Asian American scholars whose illnesses circumscribe and, in many ways, help theorize their scholarly projects. Thus, they stage, counterintuitively, the scholarly monograph—a genre committed to notions of trenchant rigor and modes of rhetoric largely shorn of affect—as the place of life writing. This insertion of the intimate, vulnerable self into the very language of critical theory, and of its rhetorical disposition of critique, puts the critical enterprise at extreme risk: the voice of the scholar-author's sentiment may come to contaminate the methodological soundness of the monograph, or, conversely, the scholars may have to vanish themselves to remain committed to the vocation of critique. Or something else might happen. What the works of Mel Chen, S. Lochlann Jain, and Lana Lin offer instead are less interventions than experiments in critical subject formation. Asian American(ist) scholars occupy a double consciousness of sorts, of a model minority fashion: keenly aware of the cultural logics that afforded Asian Americans like them access to modes of education and other forms of knowledge production, they wield the critical armature to interrogate their own formations as subjects of and to, say, institutional power. Yet, they insist, the interruption of the ill self matters, and matters crucially, for themselves surely, but also for the sake of what one might call an ethically engaged scholarship in the first place. These scholars work in their monograph memoirs to forge a complex personhood of illness, of embodiment and of ill *thought*, that offers a telos for what a criticism that takes up its own woundedness and vulnerability might do to offer not just insight but also, perhaps, something that approximates a social good.

The kernel of this book itself bears the autobiographical impulse of my own training—and learning. In the summer of 2009, I spent four hundred hours working as a chaplain intern at the Hospital of the Good Samaritan in downtown Los Angeles. Along with five other interns, I participated in the hospital's Clinical Pastoral Education (CPE) program, which credentials those who are considering careers in chaplaincy and is often required for people pursuing some form of ordination in a religious tradition. The latter applied to me; I've been an Episcopal priest since 2013. I was assigned to the oncology/medical surgery floor, though I was free to go to other units. Once a week I spent evenings on call for the hospital's emergency room. Our "work" during the summer was to reflect on our encounters in these clinical spaces—hospital rooms, hallways, cafeterias—wherever and whenever we engaged in some interaction that required emotional and spiritual reflection. Often this involved talking with patients and their families, although conversations with hospital staff were not uncommon.

The Rev. Dr. Ronald David, our CPE director, encouraged us not to follow the advice of health-care professionals who thought a patient might want to chat with a chaplain (often this request was to make a patient more compliant to medical directives), but to "enter the mystery" by asking for permission from people when I entered their rooms and to remain curious about what might unfold. I was terrified when I began, and the dread of anticipation didn't abate all summer. By the summer of 2009, I had completed a year's worth of theological training in the seminary I was attending as my educational requirement for ordination, and I found this work to be both enjoyable and familiar, given the methodological and theoretical parallels of the religious and secular humanities, despite the pretense of a firewall. But neither the readings and papers from that year, nor the experience of being a tenured scholar, of teaching, of writing, and perhaps most of all, of reading text carefully—all that training—none of it found any use when I crossed the threshold of a patient room's and asked the person lying there before me what she or he might want to talk about, to share: the man from Guam who wouldn't look me in the eye the first time I visited him but over the course of two weeks would tell me his life story—and about his experience of medical brutalization at the hospital, which accounted for his initial refusal to communicate; the young Latinx man, really a teenager, who stared blankly at a piece of paper showing that the tumor inside his skull had metastasized while his wife held him, uninterested in holding back tears; the woman from El Salvador who was convinced she had murdered her unborn child through a procedure performed by doctors because the failed pregnancy threatened to kill her; the quiet area in the emergency room cordoned off by only a curtain as a family gently caressed their elder patriarch who had died an hour earlier, a silence that belied the actual clanging of the medical devices beyond the curtain. I could go on, because the stories are legion, and like all texts, their stories are worlds.

These stories, these encounters, remain as vivid to me as I complete this book more than a decade later as they were when I experienced them in 2009. I knew then, as I was going through my brief brush with chaplaincy, that the experience of human woundedness—illness, death, and suffering—bent the shape of the story and quietly insisted, demanded, a hearing of a different sort. I was lucky that my director, Dr. David, who knew about my training in literary criticism, encouraged me to read Frank's *The Wounded Storyteller*; you will see him all over this book. Perhaps most crucial for me that summer, and in what I have tried to practice since then, was to engage in as generous a reading practice of any story I encounter and to see what happens when one is as open and vulnerable and curious about another's telling as one has the bandwidth to allow. I jettison none of the critical armature I've accumulated throughout my scholarly career, for animating the forces that underpin any text, in whatever form, is vital to see its worlding, especially its most fucked-up versions. But rigor can be—and, indeed, must be—tender. This, then, is a training and a learning of a different sort that I hope you, too, will try on.

This experience of stories turning me, stopping me cold, insisting to be heard—in effect, demanding a public ear of at least one chaplain—undergirds my insistence on the importance of the memoir genre. Memoirs, as idiosyncratic as the people who write them, are narrative actions of "participation in the public sphere."[54] Mind you, this isn't a public sphere that Jürgen Habermas would recognize; nor is it one insulated from the lashes of market forces and expectations. So, like their authors, memoirs are fragile objects, easily misunderstood or dismissed for presumed lower quality or unexamined bias or grandeurs of celebrity. But even with the rise of so many platforms for communication and communicability, such as blogs, social media, and personal websites, there is an inverse relation to the valuation of selfhood. Asian Americans strive to find themselves in U.S. society, and their constricted form of recognition is a model minority suit, off-the-rack or bespoke. People get sick and go to the doctor and are ordered to take off their clothes and slip into a gown whose openness feels universally invasive; they soon learn that they are little more than a litany of symptoms and prognoses, at risk of losing their narrative anchor and temporality. The genre of memoir provides in the act of writing, for those who have experienced the profanities of existential loss, the work of re-enchantment of the "I" in the self and of sharing this reimagined "I" with another who might be their chaplain for a time, a kind of book-length training. For some, this act of writing the memoir may be their first gesture of examining who this "I" is, because forms of able-bodiedness presumed a fixed understanding, a knowing now undone by illness, whether theirs or another's. But in either case, memoirs insist on a reading and hearing; thus, they are "act of commitments to self and others."[55] To rediscover the "I" is no easy task and offers no guarantee for identification or recognition. I hope you will honor the possibility of witness by reading beside them in their narrative journey.

This book therefore limns the incommensurabilities of reading for exposure and reading for repair. It understands that memoirs about illness and death by Asian Americans are, of course, expressions and effects of biomedical discourse and of the political economies of a medical-industrial complex. Memoirs to this extent are certainly symptomatic of the contemporary impulse to make the individual bear the burden of experiences better shared and addressed in the collective; this, of course, is neoliberalism's logic, which deputizes Asian Americans such as Julie Yip-Williams as the examples who show the rest of us how it should be done. But when bodies fail, whether those in one's professional care or one's own, they demand an accounting and a hearing that implores, begs even, at least a pause—and, I would urge, a bit longer than that—in the critical reflex. "What if we regularly upheld care not just as a bonus activity or a by-product of scholarship?" asks the musicologist and disability studies scholar William Cheng, who follows up with this equally important question: "In a world where injuries run rampant, what if care *is* the point?"[56] Even the most utopian formation can't do away with the inevitable woundedness of our bodies. So to begin to care, even love, these bodies in and of failure demands, first, that we sit and read the words that come from these bodies and the words written by those changed by these bodies. If there is any possibility to imagine an Asian American future, or a future in general, that doesn't insist on the optimization of social life as a form of extraction, and if there is an Asian American formation that can finally put the model minority to rest, it will begin when we breathe in the words of the ill and dying and let these stories change how we breathe and move through the world. A scholarly consideration of narratives about and of illness needs for its vocation to be about clearing a bit of space for this, to let such stories breathe.[57]

1

The Desification of the Doctor and the Ends of Medicine

Giving Up Mastery: The Case of Jhumpa Lahiri

In the middle of her first novel, *The Namesake* (2002), Jhumpa Lahiri's protagonist Gogol Ganguli finds himself in his girlfriend's swanky apartment, where he experiences something that one might call a teachable moment. Up to this point, the narrative has carefully traced the stories of Gogol's parents, Ashima and Ashoke, Bengali immigrants from Calcutta who have made a home in a Boston suburb and must negotiate how to instill in their U.S.-born children a sense of their Bengali origins under the quiet but relentless pull of plastic, disposable American commodity culture. Young Gogol develops a knack for simplicity: he cries when his parents tell him that, when he enters kindergarten, teachers and classmates will call him Nikhil, his "good" or public name, instead of Gogol, the intimate pet name reserved for family. Gogol rejects this multiplicity of identity and insists on being called Gogol in all his childhood spheres, only to reverse this by the time he turns eighteen, when he changes his name legally to Nikhil. By this point he loathes the name given to him by his father, which is "neither American nor Indian but of all things Russian." So it should come as no surprise to Lahiri's readers that college and graduation have Gogol pulling farther away from the centripetal orbit of immigrant desi culture that Ashima and Ashoke try so hard to maintain.

While he struggles with his identity mostly through acts of negation, those elements of Indian immigrant life he tries to gently disavow, it is when Gogol meets Maxine Ratliff, moneyed and unencumbered by any notion of cultural specificity, that he, as the narrative puts it, falls in love. But it is not just Maxine who is the object of Gogol's desire. A broader and more insidious yearning is at work when he slides into the lives of Maxine, and of Gerald and Lydia, her parents:

> Quickly, simultaneously, he falls in love with Maxine, the house, and Gerald and Lydia's manner of living, for to know her and love her is to know and love all of these things. He loves the mess that surrounds Maxine, her hundreds of things always covering her floor and her bedside table, her habit, when they are alone on the fifth floor, of not shutting the door when she goes to the bathroom. Her unkempt ways, a challenge to his increasingly minimalist taste, charm him. *He learns to love* the food she and her parents eat, the polenta and risotto, the bouillabaisse and osso buco, the meat baked in parchment paper. He comes to expect the weight of their flatware in his hands, and to keep the cloth napkin, still partially folded on his lap. *He learns* that one does not grate Parmesan cheese over pasta dishes containing seafood. *He learns* not to put wooden spoons in the dishwater, as he had mistakenly done one evening when he was helping to clean up. The nights he spends there, *he learns* to wake up earlier than he is used to, to the sound of Silas barking downstairs, wanting to be taken for his morning walk. *He learns* to anticipate, every evening, the sound of a cork emerging from a fresh bottle of wine.[1]

That Lahiri couches Gogol and Maxine's romance in terms of pedagogy shouldn't surprise, as there are several instances in the novel in which assimilation as a form of education quietly emerges for all of her Indian American characters. What is striking in this passage is not simply that it thematizes the broader cultural and racial problematic that haunts Gogol, who otherwise is socially fine—Ivy League–educated and on his way to a successful career in architecture—but that the pedagogy of assimilation comes in such minute, ordinary, corporeal, and sensory changes: the food he takes in, the hand resting on his lap *this* way, the awakening from slumber still just a little too tired, the sounds that he wants to make familiar a bit too eagerly. This is not the discipline of Bentham's panopticon but, rather, the so much more effective biopolitics of the care of the self, the cultivation of improvement in which a regime of cultural value is adopted voluntarily.

If the gentle seduction of Gogol's assimilation is the heart of Lahiri's tragedy in *The Namesake*, the ease with which Gogol falls for Maxine and all she represents is matched by the formal satisfaction of Lahiri's prose. Take, for instance, the repetition of the verb "learns," which doesn't feel repetitive, Lahiri's almost matter-of-fact description of Gogol's descent into the doldrums of whiteness that is interrupted only by the sudden and unexpected death of his father, Ashoke, from a massive heart attack. Perhaps more than any other contemporary Asian American author, Lahiri has honed what Min Hyoung Song calls a "mastery of form" that is at once both unselfconscious and deliberate.[2] Her deployment of free indirect discourse in this passage formally mirrors the pedagogy of assimilation: not by rote or by violence, but by the simple ingestion of things into one's own so that the boundaries of self and environment, thought and action, are indistinguishable, just as incorporating white culture into Gogol's subjectivity comes to feel as expected as the feeling of love itself. He finds beauty in his newfound love for white culture, which Lahiri composes in beautifully wrought sentences that her mostly white reviewers adore.

Perhaps this is why, while there is no shortage of celebrated authors of South Asian descent within the reading West—think Salman Rushdie, Arundhati Roy, Amitav Ghosh, even V. S. Naipaul—"none has been honored by the American literati as magnanimously as Jhumpa Lahiri," as Lavina Dhingra and Floyd Cheung have suggested.[3] Highlighting not only the Pulitzer Prize she won for her first book, but also the numerous book clubs that feature her work, the adoption of her books and stories (through venues such as the *New Yorker*) in high school and college courses, and the anthologizing of her stories in "best of" collections, Dhingra and Cheung recognize "Lahiri's importance as a complex, transnational contemporary writer and . . . her works' remarkable aesthetic quality." They ask pointedly in their volume dedicated to answering their rhetorical question, "Why is Lahiri's writing so successful among multiple audiences?"[4] To this they echo Lev Grossman's observation that Lahiri's aesthetics make her readers realize that "we're way more interested in Bengali immigrants than we thought we were."[5] Readers thus *learn to love* Bengali immigrants because they are crafted in Lahiri's breathless prose, readers taught about other lives by someone whose mastery of form makes them desire this South Asian American pedagogy.

And yet just as Gogol will suffer a huge cost in his affection for the white culture embodied in Maxine's family, in the form of a futurity in which his South Asian American family is disassembled, so, too, does the widely and deeply held readerly affect for Lahiri's prose bear a burden for the author. She expresses this burden first in an essay in the *New Yorker* in 2015 titled "Teach Yourself Italian" and later in the book-length memoir *In Other Words*

(2015).[6] "For practically my whole life," Lahiri writes in the essay, "English has represented a consuming struggle, a wrenching conflict, a continuous sense of failure that is the source of almost all my anxiety. It has represented a culture that had to be mastered, interpreted. I was afraid that it meant a break between me and my parents. English denotes a heavy, burdensome aspect of my past. I'm tired of it. And yet I was in love with it. I became a writer in English."[7] It's not hard to see in this passage a deep resonance between Lahiri's vexed love for English, a love so strong that she feels the responsibility to master it, and Gogol's fraught love for Maxine, which means to "know and love all these things." It is this special burden of exceptional performance borne by the "children of 1965," whom Min Hyoung Song observes "have been lovingly and anxiously fantasized into existence over the past several decades."[8] But being the object of fantasy is, as Lahiri puts it, tiring. So she abandons English, moves to Italy, and begins to write, haltingly, in Italian: "I don't recognize the person who is writing in this diary, in this new, approximate language. But I know that it's the most genuine, most vulnerable part of me."[9] Precision gives way to approximation, mastery to vulnerability; it is as if, in writing so exactingly to help her readers delight in their interest in her Bengali characters, Lahiri teaches—or, rather, learns—how to be interesting once more to herself through Italian, a language from which she feels exiled even though it was never originally hers.

It's important to note here that, while Lahiri's literary story—of her almost universally acknowledged mastery of English writing; the ways that language so determines her deepest sense of affect in such fraught ways; her capacity to make South Asian American lives, including her own, interesting to so many—may be exemplary, it is by no means exceptional. The Subcontinent's postcolonial history has made its diasporic writers among the best known and best regarded of its cultural effects, as South Asian diasporic writers teach the Anglophone world how to write in English anew. Lahiri's work resonates all the more with her readers because, as an American, she departs significantly from many other contemporary U.S. writers, formed in what Mark McGurl calls the "Program Era," a period that we have not really left, whose works serve more as "testaments to the continuing interest of literary forms as objects of a certain kind of professional research."[10] Lahiri's work, by contrast, doesn't require a doctorate to enjoy; her prose makes students of lay readers. What seems so not much new but refreshing in Lahiri's works is a kind of literary pedagogy. Just as she has her readers witness how Gogol learns the intimacies of assimilation, Lahiri teaches her readers how to fall in love with Bengali life.

Falling for Your Brown Doctor:
The Aftermath of 1965

Something analogous is happening in U.S. cultures of medicine, particularly insofar as medicine is represented through various forms of narrative to represent the myriad encounters physicians and other health-care workers have with people who become their patients. In the last two decades of the twentieth century and well into this century, South Asian American physicians have not only populated hospitals, clinics, and medical research centers across the country; they have also taken up what one might call an outsize role in the public dissemination of medicine and its cultures. And like Lahiri's reach toward general readers, South Asian American physician writers do not reach colleagues in academic medical journals but, instead, serve as principal medical authorities to a notably lay readership. We might say that that South Asian American physicians in the United States take up a form of pedagogy through their writing and, in doing so, have made Americans more interested in medicine than they thought they were. And yet, as we see in this chapter, it is when these South Asian American physicians reach a level of clinical and narrative mastery in which theirs are considered the ideal form of the physician memoir that something altogether uncanny emerges. It begins with a twinge of suspicion and doubt and continues apace as the South Asian American physician wins over more and more readers and patients: a narrative revelation that clinical erudition highlights medicine's event horizon, its limit and its end, beyond which—they realize—all bodies ultimately fail.

A generation ago, it would have been risible to imagine people with surnames such as Gawande, Verghese, Mukherjee, Kalanithi, Murthy, Jauhar, and Gupta as the paragons of U.S. medicine, yet today they are practically household names, given that almost all of them are not only practicing physicians but telegraph this clinical work through their narrative representation of it. What accounts for the desification of medical literary celebrity? To answer this question, we must turn first to the historical and the sociological.

It is very hard to overstate the historic importance of the 1965 Immigration Act in enabling the emergence of this cohort of South Asian American doctors. In moving from a restrictive policy based almost entirely on national origins toward one based on labor needs in the United States and employment preferences of American companies (as well as family unification), the Immigration and Nationality Act of 1965 (also known as the Hart-Celler Act) catalyzed the migration of millions who came to the United States with high levels of education and professionalization in sectors that required (and still need) people with such skill sets, engineering and health care among them. It is, of course, this act that enabled (South) Asian America's half-century of explosive growth, something that a previous generation would have thought unimaginable. Prior to 1965, South Asian migrants were subjected to an exclusionary immigration regime based primarily on race and national origins, the underpinnings of which were the Page Act of 1875, which barred Chinese women from entering the United States to stave off the moral panic of widespread prostitution, and, later, the 1882 Chinese Exclusion Act, which barred a specific racial group from entry to the United States. After the Supreme Court upheld the Exclusion Act and, more generally, Congress's plenary power to decide who would be allowed into the United States, the expansion of exclusion and restriction continued apace throughout most of the first half of the twentieth century. So almost as soon as the first group of a few hundred (mostly) men from the state of Punjab arrived in California in the early twentieth century, anti-Indian exclusion leagues formed alongside anti-Japanese and anti-Korean versions, whose political pressure moved Congress to pass the Immigration Act of 1917 (also known as the Asiatic Barred Zone Act) and the National Origins Act of 1924. The former restricted immigration from regions of the world as far east as most of China (and all of Southeast Asia and the Indian Subcontinent) and as far west as modern-day Turkey, while the latter established severe quotas based on a potential migrant's national origin. Immigration restriction is perhaps the crudest form of biopolitical management, as it is the most obvious in highlighting what constitutes an idealized national subject by simply shutting out a nation's undesirables, and the effects of the 1917 and 1924 laws were quite stark on the South Asian American community. By 1960, the year of the last U.S. Census before the passage of the 1965 act, the official count of South Asians stood at a paltry 12,296.[11]

Meanwhile, on the Subcontinent, economic and demographic changes matched the political transformation of the postcolonial nations that emerged after Independence and Partition in 1947. "By the mid-1960s," Sanjoy Chakravorty, Devesh Kapur, and Nirvikar Singh write, "India had created a small network of good-quality institutions of higher education. . . . However, as India's economy stagnated during the 1960s and 1970s, the demand for the highly-skilled graduates of these institutions was tepid."[12] While a surplus of India's educated but unemployable elites constituted the push factor for migrants, the pull factor to come to the United States took the form of Hart-Celler and the pressures that led to its passage. As Eram Alam has deftly highlighted, one of the precipitating factors that led to the passage of the act, even in the face of ongoing concern and even hostility toward the idea of allowing immigration from regions that had long been seen as full of undesirable and unassimilable peoples, was the reportage of the perceived and real "doctor shortage" in the United States at the very moment that India was swelling with graduating medical students.[13] Thanks to a combination of the American Medical Association's firm grip on medical credentialing standards,[14] rising costs of medical education, and, later, the drafting of physicians in the service of the war in Vietnam and President Lyndon Johnson's War on Poverty (one of whose pillars would become the expansion of health care through Medicare and Medicaid), journalistic coverage of the shortage crisis, of the lack of physicians at the same time demand for medical service was increasing, helped push lawmakers to see the value in shedding national origin as a criterion for eligibility to enter and, importantly, work in the United States. Congressman Emanuel Celler, the sponsor of the House version of the bill, said in a speech on the floor during the debate over the bill's passage in 1964, "Shall we not as a nation have the means whereby we can choose freely from all corners of the earth the talents and the skills we need and not limit our choice because one man of genius was born 5 miles east or south of an arbitrarily traced boundary?"[15] This would be the way to convince skeptical colleagues to ditch the obsession with race, Alam notes, and to find a new and better way to preserve American exceptionalism.[16]

Among these "geniuses" were, of course, the physicians the United States needed critically and immediately, and it is this group that made up a broad swath of the early wave of post-1965 immigrants to the United States. Between 1965 and 1979, twelve thousand Indians migrated to the United States. Almost half of them came with professional—often, medical—degrees, but almost all of them were "very accomplished individuals who gained legal entry based on their education and skills."[17] These "early movers" of the post-1965 era (Chakravorty and colleagues' phrase) would be joined by far more South Asian immigrants after 1980, many of whom would secure employment through the H-1B visa program, but even as the initial "crisis" of the doctor shortage waned in the early 1980s, the use of foreign physician labor is now a durable feature of post-1965 U.S. life. "Since 1965," Alam writes, "immigration has become a requisite method of procuring adequate physician labour in the United States, resulting in foreign physicians constituting at least a quarter of the labour force. No longer a temporary solution, FMGs [foreign medical graduates] have become an indispensable labour force marshalled to provide services in certain areas where doctor shortage crises have become a regular feature of the health care system."[18] And while there are significant sectors of the South Asian community who come to the United States with far fewer material and human capital resources, those who make up the community's working poor, the preponderance of highly educated and skilled students and workers continues: the 1990 Census shows that Asian Indians held the highest percentage of those with bachelor's degrees or higher (48.7 percent versus 17.6 percent, U.S. average) and those occupied in "managerial or professional specialty" (43.6 percent versus 26.4 percent, U.S. average) within Asian America.[19] In 1965, the United States needed South Asian American physicians. It was a long half-century courtship—and long enough for Americans to fall in love with their brown doctors.

Guru Interregnum: Deepak Chopra and Sanjay Gupta

Yet demography alone can't account for how South Asian American physicians would enter the cultural imaginations of Americans as disseminators of medical culture, along with serving as dispensers of health care. For this pivot from clinic to media, practice to discourse, we might begin, actually, with a figure who has not yet been mentioned but remains South Asian America's most popular and most contested physician, someone whose fame emerged because of his pivot away from (if not his deeper disavowal of) allopathic medicine. Deepak Chopra attended the All India Institute of Medical Sciences in New Delhi, graduating in 1969. Then, like thousands of other FMGs from South Asia, he immigrated to the United States, where he interned in New Jersey and completed residencies in internal medicine and endocrinology in the Boston area. But, of course, it is not his medical credentials for which he well known (though, crucially, he maintains a medical license; more on this in a moment). Rather, he is known for his philosophical and practical commitments to his own form of alternative medicine, a cultural, nonspecific version of Ayurvedic medicine that Chopra has called "quantum healing." Chopra's career figuratively and literally crossed paths with another popular South Asian figure in the United States, Maharishi Mahesh Yogi. Founder of the India-based Spiritual Regeneration Movement and a major figure in the Transcendental Meditation (TM) movement, he is famed for attracting celebrity followers such as the Beatles, David Lynch, Elizabeth Taylor, and Mia Farrow. Chopra's meeting with the Maharishi in 1985 convinced him to abandon his private practice and leave New England Memorial Hospital to establish an Ayurvedic center on behalf of TM. Chopra would remain a spokesperson for TM for eight years; the two parted ways in 1993 after the Maharishi accused Chopra of trying to usurp him as the guru, while Chopra feared that an ongoing connection to TM might hurt his chances of making Ayurvedic medicine legitimate in the eyes of his biomedical colleagues.

In her study of the Maharishi, Jane Iwamura argues that such "Oriental Monks" are circumscribed by a strict script of persona to maintain their aura with Western audiences: "A certain degree of foreignness and a strict divide between East and West emerge as significant prerequisites for recognition of an individual as an Oriental Monk figure. When an Asian spiritual leader crosses that divide, like Mahesh, his behavior becomes suspect, and his image subsequently tainted."[20] To keep Americans and other Westerners in an Orientalist thrall, Oriental Monks must continue to traffic in notions of Asian anachronism, which, in turn, affords them a spirituality that is now lost to the West, beset as it is by capitalism and attendant materialism. So Iwamura finds that part of the reason for waning of the Maharishi's legitimacy over time had to do in part with his seeming ease with the trappings of the West: photographs of the Maharishi flying in a helicopter or talking on the phone served to heighten skepticism that TM was more style than religion, more scene than spirit.[21] The very persona that cast the Maharishi as a figure of spiritual wisdom for so many made him vulnerable to charges of hucksterism by his skeptics, who were eager to point out how much he stood to gain economically by his popularity. By contrast, Chopra seems to have arrived at his celebrity as a South Asian American "guru" in reverse, trained as he was in Western biomedicine in postcolonial India and the United States before pivoting to his form of Ayurvedic practices. Alam argues that this biomedical training "legitimated him as an authoritative figure on matters of sickness and health. Only after that validation could Chopra reintegrate the cultural practices of India back into his healing lexicon and repertoire in a manner that was ahistorical and apolitical."[22] If what is required of the Oriental Monk is a firm boundary between the world he inhabits and the modern world the rest of us live in, for Chopra the contemporary South Asian American healer mandates that he continue to hold a passport into the annals of Western medicine, a blend, as it were, of East and West.

Vijay Prashad rightly critiques Chopra's enterprise as a form of "New Age Orientalism," which follows a genealogy far beyond Chopra and the Maharishi of what he calls "sly *babas* and other gurus" that goes as far back as the turn of the twentieth century. What binds each of these figures is the ability of the "gurus" to turn social problems into matters that require individuated responses. "The individual," Prashad observes of Chopra's core idea, "must ignore social connectedness and revel in interiority. Interior knowledge (consciousness) is the source of reality for Chopra; therefore it is in this realm that change must be effected."[23] Turning to Chopra's version of Ayurvedic "healing," Prashad likewise finds fault in his isolation of the "mind-body complex" to individual praxis rather than addressing the social origins of many human afflictions that his practice is meant to address: "By reducing the body to the individual body, Chopra can ignore irrefutable social factors that produce social problems, and he can locate the etiology of the problems of the mind-body complex (the individual), which is all that then needs to be treated. Chopra draws from a vast corpus of ancient wisdom on healing, but he make[s] of the corpus marketable indulgences that are sold to a harassed elite and middle-class who want to relax but not to change what makes them tense."[24] But this deep and critical review of Chopra's thinking hinges on a view of contemporary health care that Prashad and Chopra share—namely, "the crisis in allopathic medicine and the U.S. healthcare system."[25] Highlighting the epistemological flaw in the allopathic approach—its tendency to think of the ailing body instrumentally and divide it into discrete "entities to study them in detail" (which mirrors the tendency in medicine toward ever more forms of specialization); its inability to address the psychosocial context of people with ailments and woundedness; and its profound disparities in the distribution and quality of health toward different communities—Prashad asserts (and thus quietly concurs with Chopra) that the "medical-industrial complex cannot hope to be an agent of healing."[26]

In *Ageless Body, Timeless Mind: The Quantum Alternative to Growing Old* (1993), which sold 100,000 copies in a single day after he appeared on *The Oprah Winfrey Show*, Chopra insists that consciousness and awareness are all that are required to stop the process of aging and, by extension, mortality: "There is no biochemistry outside awareness; every cell in your body is totally aware of how you think and feel about yourself. Once you accept that fact, the whole illusion of being victimized by a mindless, randomly degenerating body falls away."[27] Such sentences aren't atypical in this or any of Chopra's other books, of which there are, to date, more than eighty. The durability of the Chopra brand and the fact that his popularity has enabled him to establish a for-profit center and a nonprofit foundation, and secured significant personal wealth since that time, surely infuriates his critics and skeptics, of which there are many.[28] His continued cultural significance and material success signal that Chopra, like Oriental Monks before him, serves as an "*ideological caregiver* who gains recognition by helping dominant white Americans gain spiritual insight and, often, political mission as they work out the meaning of their existence in modern life."[29] To this one might add that, in the context of health care, Chopra himself provides his followers with an aesthetic form, the figuration as a South Asian American with a medical license who leads them away from the hospital and its attendant industry. His attraction for so many is symptomatic of a deep crisis that U.S. biomedicine has faced for more than a generation, which is actually a Gordian knot of crises: the material crisis of health care's exponential rising costs and its unequal distribution of care and coverage; the existential crisis of its inability to improve people's quality of life, despite advances in medical and pharmaceutical technology; and the phenomenological crisis of deteriorating relations between patients and health-care providers, to name just the most transparent. Chopra's Oriental Monk with a medical degree represents, then, a racial aesthetic to mobilize a renunciatory politics whose rhetoric of wellness, abundance, and even immortality points to a severe cynicism about what contemporary biomedicine has wrought.

Despite the consistency of charges of hucksterism from his critics, Chopra's message of prosperity, spontaneous healing, and even immortality— what disability studies might call a hypercharged version of ableism—remains durable. And in the popular imagination it remains transferable, especially if the South Asian healing "guru" can optimize his reach by the moral armature of biomedical science and the digestibility of a sanitized racialized figure of, say, Sanjay Gupta, who since 2003 has served as "chief medical correspondent" for the cable television news channel CNN. Trained as a neurosurgeon and institutionally based at Grady Memorial Hospital in Atlanta (where CNN is conveniently headquartered), Gupta certainly looks the part: on television he appears well-coiffed, in perfect-fitting, likely bespoke suits with occasional B-roll presenting him in surgical scrubs. His racial brownness might risk his sliding into the kind of skeptical reception that Chopra receives from the medical community and audiences not inclined to quantum healing, but the auditory mitigates the threat of shared racial visuality. Whereas Chopra's accent reinforces him as an Oriental Monk in the vein of the Maharishi, Gupta's midwestern American accent serves to shore up the thoroughly model-minoritized public identity, buttressed by elite medical authority, that has made him incontrovertibly a well-received journalist in news related to health care.[30] Gupta's presentational ease also helps in advancing his particular function as a South Asian American authority: while Chopra's late twentieth-century emergence indexes a general crisis of faith in contemporary medicine's ability to deliver forms of health care that care for its recipients, Gupta's popular arrival in the early twenty-first century represents the use of the South Asian American as medical apologist. The latter telegraphs a latter-day optimism and a gentle form of paternalism of a prior era, retooled for contemporary reception. Gupta is, and perhaps remains, U.S. medicine's unapologetic cheerleader, almost immune to the collective misery into which Chopra's message has tapped.

In addition to the conveniently captured footage of his own medical heroism—Gupta famously performed emergency surgery on an injured U.S. marine while he was imbedded with a unit during the invasion of Iraq in 2003, a procedure that was broadcast on CNN—Gupta has turned to writing to consolidate this vision of medical as progressive and salvific.[31] He is the author of three books—including, most recently, a novel—but it is the titles of his two works of nonfiction and this genre's proximity to facticity that I highlight: *Chasing Life: New Discoveries in the Search for Immortality to Help You Age Less Today* (2008) and *Cheating Death: The Doctors and Medical Miracles That Are Saving Lives against All Odds* (2009). The titles make clear that Gupta is deeply invested in the discourse of medical heroism, the doctor as protagonist and figure of absolute rescue—the role doctors play within the rubric of what the scholar Arthur Frank calls modernist medicine. By extension, the role that the ill person plays in this drama is that of the patient, whose obligation in seeking care is thus to surrender her narrative to the story that the physician gets to tell. "The ill person," Frank writes, "not only agrees to follow physical regimens that are prescribed; she also agrees, tacitly but with no less implication, to tell her story in medical terms. . . . The physician becomes the spokesperson for the disease, and the ill person's stories come to depend heavily on repetition of what the physician has said."[32] As a spokesperson for disease, Gupta is unabashed in telling a progressive story about medicine and its capacity to, as he puts it in *Cheating Death*, "shift the line between life and death."[33] He frames the book with the story of Zeyad Barazanji, a Syrian American academic who suffers a heart attack and by all accounts should be dead. But thanks to experimental technologies and new therapies, which include therapeutic hypothermia, induced hibernation, and new cardiopulmonary resuscitation (CPR) techniques, as well as unrelated practices such as fetal surgery, Gupta is able to end the book proudly with an account of meeting Barazanji at his home in New York as they prepare to take a walk at dusk on an autumn day. As they walk to Barazanji's favorite spot, Gupta closes the book with this image: "[Barazanji] closed his eyes. Death was nowhere to be seen."[34]

Indeed, Gupta is at pains to use these anecdotes as evidence not only of medical heroism but also of medicine's inherent futurity, a utopian biopolitics to which we all should assent. Early in his narrative Gupta offers a distillation of this progressive narrative:

The practice of medicine is changing constantly. The innovation isn't always for the better—ask one of the women who took thalidomide in the 1960s to ward off morning sickness. And innovation is never easy—most of the first heart transplant patients died within hours or days of their transplant. But the next round of transplants went better, and then better, and today thousands of heart transplant patients live rich lives because of the bold pioneers of the 1950s and 1960s and their brave subjects. What I have learned is that this cycle—desperation, desperate measure, apparent miracle, insight, common practice—shifts the line in the sand. That's how medicine moves forward.[35]

Here, then, is the South Asian American doctor whom American readers implicitly trust rehearsing the progressive temporality of medicine as unqualified triumph. The "1950s and 1960s," during which experimentation by "bold pioneers" took place, is also the era of medical paternalism; physicians and other researchers would never again enjoy such unreserved submission to authority by their patients. But even in this summary statement on biomedical triumph and its seemingly unrelenting forward movement, Gupta must acknowledge, even as he quickly dismisses, the horror of medical fallacy. Thalidomide, a drug marketed to counter the effects of morning sickness and at one point sold as an over-the-counter medication, had the terrible effect of malforming fetal limbs. Ten thousand children were born with significant disabilities, and only half of them survived infancy. And there are the hundreds of transplant patients—the "brave subjects"—who had to die before others could live "rich lives." Thus, we see even in this attempt to narrate medicine's biopolitical triumph its necropolitical foundations: for each and every example that Gupta champions, thousands of others don't survive. This fatal redemption story, the necropolitical underpinnings of Gupta's biopolitics of flourishing, is thus premised on patients' surrendering to the absolute agency of physicians, for their own good. What haunts Gupta's optimism parallels the haunting of our South Asian American model minority physician tasked with leading America to utopian health care: the South Asian American physician compels submission to medical authority, knowledge, and technology to maintain the narrative of patient restitution and recovery for a few, even as many others are sacrificed. But the real story is that his narratives speak finally and fundamentally to the necropolitical dimensions of the biopolitical flourishing not of patients at all, but of the South Asian American physician. Indeed, for all of his invocations of melodrama in the patient stories that he tells in *Cheating Death*, there is a remarkable lack of self or personhood in the patients. Really, the patients are little more than the ill, diseased, or injured bodies on whom medical "miracles" are performed.

In many ways, Chopra and Gupta suffer a similar disposition: that of the South Asian American male authority whose vision of health care is so total, so complete, that it can brook no possibility of ambivalence for his mode. Neither can traffic in the realism of the inevitability of finitude and the affective messiness that suffuses the experiences of illness and death—for those suffering maladies and those tasked with treating them. Chopra and Gupta both rely on a profoundly monadic understanding of their respective narratives of health care, both of which promise restoration to health of sick bodies. We might even call their writings a sub-subgenre of speculative fictive nonfiction, a health-care utopianism that must banish those shadow stories that don't result in normative bodily flourishing. But realism is called for, both in the clinic and on the page. Disability studies' central insight and insistence that non-able-bodied people can and should be central producers of the meaning of their bodies means that, at minimum, a medical narrative must at least gesture to the dialogic dimensions and the multiplicity of bodyminds at play in clinical encounters.[36] If Americans are to learn something from South Asian American medical authority, and if there is to be a chance for post-1965 South Asian American medical narrative pedagogy to take hold, it behooves these physicians to learn something about the people on whose bodies they exercise their medical skills. What is needed, then, are less the speculative genres of Chopra and Gupta than a realist substratum that witnesses and acknowledges the fraught and the vulnerable inherent in attention to ill and disabled people, even if in the service of leading their readers to more hopeful imaginaries. The United States wanted from its South Asian American figures nothing less than a narrative roadmap for a health-care future worth living into.

Desi Southern Gothic: Abraham Verghese

Abraham Verghese's first memoir, *My Own Country* (1994), which chronicled his medical sojourn in eastern Tennessee at the height of the AIDS epidemic, narrates the post-1965 journey of physicians to otherwise unlikely places for South Asian immigrants. By the 1980s, the arrival of South Asian FMGs coincided with deleterious effects of decades of deindustrialization and underinvestment in the U.S. economy and policy withdrawals at almost all levels of the government so that these doctors served a new social function: to work in those places that their U.S.-born white counterparts would largely abandon. "[T]he once grand county hospitals were sliding inexorably, like the cities themselves, into critical states," reflects Verghese, and the largely uninsured and indigent patients consigned to these spaces were met by medical staff that looked like him. "An inevitable accompaniment to this scene of a city hospital under siege was the sight of foreign physicians. The names of these doctors—names such as Srivastava, Patel, Khan, Iqbal, Hussein, Venkateswara, Menon—bore no resemblance to those of the patients being served or the physicians who supervised them."[37] The presence of immigrant physicians from the Subcontinent practicing medicine in urban poor communities of color has its corollary in poor, rural, white communities such as the one that Verghese would work in for the bulk of his narrative. Like his colleagues in the large cities, the physicians at the Johnson City Medical Center were so overwhelmingly South Asian that, Verghese recounts, the non–South Asian emergency room staff could discern Madrasi from Gujarati accents.[38] While he later contrasts himself from what he views as the "parochial" ways of the South Asian community and its interaction with the locals, Verghese situates himself as part of this medical diaspora, as just one of the thousands enlisted and enticed to arrive and work and live in the places that other American physician colleagues had abandoned, not unlike the ways that immigrants employ similar chain migration techniques. "Meanwhile, year by year," he writes, "more foreign physicians, recruited by the same word-of-mouth that brings fresh blood to the newspaper kiosks, motels, gas stations, taxis fleets, restaurants and wholescale groceries of America, were completing their training in American urban war zones and moving into these rural havens."[39]

In many ways, Verghese's framing of his story as an unexceptional, mundane one about immigration and eventual incorporation into this rural southern community highlights a crucial dimension of the Hart-Celler Act that has long been socially felt but rarely verbalized explicitly. If the fact that there are currently more than forty thousand physicians of South Asian descent in the United States (or one in every twenty doctors) lends itself to the controlling image of the South Asian American community as a model minority formation, then we might ask what function the 1965 act might have played in such a formation. Disability studies scholars have long suggested that U.S. immigration policy has been deeply interconnected with what constitutes an ideal subject, not only in terms of race or national origin, but also in terms of the relative social value through economic productivity a potential migrant might bring if allowed entry or, conversely, rejected. Cynthia Wu notes that Congress's first major action on immigration in 1882 was designed to establish categories that justified the exclusion of people based on disability just before the passage of the Chinese Exclusion Act; called, generically, the Immigration Act of 1882, the law sought to bar from the United States any potential immigrant who was a "lunatic, idiot, or any person unable to take care of himself or herself without becoming a public charge."[40] The timing of the two laws' passage places race and disability as at least proximal, if not interconnected. Indeed, Jay Timothy Dolmage argues as much when he writes that immigration policy and its rhetoric historically have depended on the flawed "science" of eugenics to link racial status with some form of bodily degeneracy, both of which are forms of social devaluation of certain bodies that warrant exclusion from North America.[41]

In this light, we might, as scholars such as Vijay Prashad have cautioned, view the 1965 act or its consequences not in purely celebratory ways but, rather, as part of an ongoing continuum linking immigration, race, and the kinds of bodies the United States desires. Prashad avers that Hart-Celler signaled little more than a transformation in "state selectivity": crafting policy to select "preferred" migrants based on employment preference produced a demography of South Asians heavily skewed toward people and households with high levels of capital, material and cultural.[42] Built into this immigration act, of mandating a particular desirable immigrant because he or she is normatively and predictably productive, is a form of ableism. Tobin Siebers has called this the "ideology of ability," which he defines as the "baseline by which humaneness is determined, setting the measure of body and mind that gives or denies human status to individual persons."[43] The ideology of ability is pervasive, baked into the system and culture of the United States, "despite," Siebers continues, "how imbricated it may be in our thinking and practices, and despite how little we notice its patterns, authority, contradictions, and influence as a result."[44]

"The ideology of ability," Siebers summarizes, "is at its simplest the preference for able-bodiedness."[45] Thus, while pre-1965 immigration policy's focus was to manufacture able-bodiedness by restricting those the United States viewed as composed of inferior bodies, we might view the 1965 Immigration Act as a public policy expression of its converse: the championing of the ideology of ability by pulling in those viewed as desirable, over, and sometimes against, those within the United States viewed as less so.[46] Notwithstanding the persistence of opponents of mass immigration to the United States, there is in the discourse of those who champion immigration reform to enable a more porous and generous policy to admitting immigrants a tendency to highlight the relative economic benefits immigrants bring to the United States. We might thus view the arrival of South Asian American professionals as a material effect and expression of the prolonged attachment to the ideology of ability via immigration policy. And the emergence of an Asian/South Asian American cohort of physicians as an expression of post-

1965 state selection has long-lasting repercussions: just as the historical figure of the Asian American as model minority has deleteriously affected public policy toward vulnerable groups, especially other groups of color, the (South) Asian American as physician produces a set of social relationships in which Asian Americans become complicit in the creation of the contemporary patient, subjected to discourses and technologies of the medical industry. To this extent, South Asian American physicians are therefore deeply engaged in biopolitical management, as well as the stories that are valorized or minimized, or even excluded, from such management.

It is not simply, then, that South Asian American physicians such as Verghese are viewed as model minority figures in their respective communities, though he alludes to the general acknowledgment by the local community in Johnson City that the doctors are well regarded: "They developed reputations as sound physicians."[47] Rather, Verghese's presence as a participant in the medical diaspora allows his readers to view him as performing the capacities of the model minority physician, a form of autoethnography that enables us to see what a "sound physician" looks like and does. After establishing his authority to observe and develop social meaning out of his thick descriptions of the South Asian physician community; the contrasts between Boston, where he worked on a fellowship in infectious diseases, and the southern white culture of eastern Tennessee (whose overt anti-Blackness is noted but tellingly not commented on by Verghese); hospital culture; and the lush vegetation of rural Appalachia—all designed to demonstrate Verghese's observational skills and his attention to detail—we are introduced as readers to his first AIDS "case" in the character of Gordon, the sick brother of Essie, a former nursing colleague. Before examining Gordon, Verghese likens his approach to the inferential capacities of the famed fictional detective Sherlock Holmes by modeling the granularity of his attention toward the patient:

> As I interviewed [Gordon], I instinctively sized him up, trying to pick out as many clues as possible to who he was and to his condition. The patient encounter is traditionally divided into the history and the physical. But in actual fact, the examination begins the moment patients enter the room. One is alert to whether their hands are cold or warm and sweaty (which could indicate hypothyroidism or hyperthyroidism). One notes whether they are dressed shabbily or with glaring mistakes such as mismatched socks or clothing inappropriate for the season, a sign of dementia or delirium. . . . To me the history and the physical are the epitome of the internist's skill, our equivalent of the surgeon's operating room. Like Sherlock Holmes—a character based

on a superb clinician, Dr. Bell—the good internist should miss no clue, and should make the correct inference from the clues provided.[48]

The work of the "sound physician" or "good internist" centers on the doctor's ability to "miss no clue" that the patient might reveal, the physician performing nothing less than a totalizing clinical gaze. For Verghese, sizing up Gordon and his other patients is less an expression of Holmesian detachment or Foucauldian authority in relation to knowledge of the patient's body than an expression of his commitment as a physician to his patient, an act of intimacy and solidarity that is the highest expression of doctoring as a form of human attachment. It is this level of detailed observation that forms the pinnacle of patient care, from which Verghese would eventually build his career. Verghese holds himself and his medical practice as a model for the kind of relationality physicians should have with their patients and in doing so secures the rightful place for South Asian American physicians in the landscape of post-1965 U.S. culture, in medicine and writ large.

Rajini Srikanth exquisitely reads *My Own Country* as a memoir that thematizes Verghese's extraordinary gifts of observation that, paradoxically, are the result of his status as an immigrant who "inverts the figure of the immigrant-as-outsider to portray himself as the doctor who, despite his foreign-ness, is privy to the inner secrets of the land he enters."[49] Verghese's inquisitiveness highlights the subjunctive qualities of the South Asian American physician as a figure who holds an abiding interest in the stories of his patients "for their own sake." "The anecdotes they told me," he continues, "lingered in my mind and became the way I identified them. Most of these stories I kept in my head. Some I recorded in a journal that I kept faithfully and that became very important to me as time went on."[50] Here we see, as in the case of his ability to perceive "clues" to a patient's history of illness, Verghese's desire not only to abide with his patients' stories but, more crucially, to take them in as his own, to record his patients' stories in the genre linked with intimate writing: the journal. So while the act and art of observation and listening have terrifically important clinical implications, to achieve diagnostic success, such attention as a form of empathy takes on ethical and aesthetic dimensions.

That Verghese marries ethical empathy with exacting diagnostic sensitivities through the mode of writing—turning clinical and ethical dimensions into aesthetic practice—is especially significant given that this is precisely what (South) Asian American immigrants are not supposed to do. Here I take up the work of Christopher Fan, whose exploration of post-1965 Asian American fiction deftly considers C. P. Snow's "two cultures" argument in

1959: that modern Western cultures were cleaving into two separate realms—namely, the "arts" and the "sciences." Fan suggests that coterminous with the preponderance, even overrepresentation, of Asian Americans (particularly immigrants) in scientific and technical fields of employment is a dearth of Asian Americans engaging in the arts and humanities. "The widespread decision of these 'Children of 1965,'" Fan writes, "to eschew aesthetic pursuits—like writing fiction—in favor of more pragmatic and professionally secure technical training reveals a link between post-1965 immigration priorities and specific modes of the 'model minority' stereotype that . . . correspond to specific literary forms."[51] To this extent, Verghese's memoir represents an aesthetic, formal solution to the problem of the two cultures, for here we observe a member of this scientific professional community who can not only traffic in it but excel at it, to the general recognition and adulation of the arts culture in which Asian Americans are not expected to engage. The memoir becomes the means through which his professional skills render him not as mere technical automaton but, rather, as a protagonist with deep interiority and affection for his patients. Verghese himself gestures to the imperative toward the autobiographical form when, in a feature story about *My Own Country* around the time of its publication, he talks about the inadequacy of relegating his experience with AIDS patients in scholarly journals of epidemiology. The journalist Margalit Fox writes, "Dr. Verghese wrote an academic paper describing this previously undocumented epidemiology. But he knew his scientific account couldn't fully convey what he'd experienced in Johnson City. 'It neglected the stories,' he remarked. 'Not just my patients, but my own transformation from being someone who was—I wouldn't say "homophobic," but "homo-ignorant." It took the tragedy of this disease to get me to know gay men.'"[52] Scientific writing and its culture would not suffice to tell the full story of his medical sojourn with the ill and dying men and women of Johnson City; it would take a South Asian American physician who could bring arts and science together as a single subject and through the form of the subject's self-story that a compelling medical authority, fully vested in humanism, might be fashioned.

The Physician as Ethnographer as Essayist: An Excursus with Oliver Sacks

Lisa Diedrich reads Verghese's memoir as an example of a physician "becoming patient"—that is, how his encounter with people with AIDS informed different notions of "identity, empathy, and desire" from what he had learned in medical school or what he was supposed to learn in conventional medical practice. To become patient as a physician finds its analogy in the field of anthropology, for whom its best ethnographic practitioners somehow metabolize the community under study to know its vernacular from the inside, as it were. Verghese's insistence on highlighting the patient as a story, and not simply as a set of symptoms that require mere clinical observation for diagnosis, was not novel in 1994, when *My Own Country* was published. Suzanne Poirier's study of more than forty memoirs by physicians about their medical education begins with an anonymized autobiography in 1965; one of the common features of these memoirs, as in Verghese's, was a deep concern over a physician's capacity to empathize with her or his patients.[53] The medical corollary of Snow's "two cultures" has been well known in educational and clinical circles. But the author whose career most significantly resonated with Verghese, and who worked hard to resolve the problem of the bifurcation of the biomedical/biomechanical and the humanistic/psychosocial, was none other than Oliver Sacks, who, by 1994, had already written five books over more than two decades chronicling the stories of his patients (and one about himself), most of whom suffered from neurological disease. Sacks's many detractors would regard his writings—including those he would subsequently compose until his death in 2015—as little more than expositions of a narcissistic physician who exploited his patients' experience to advance a career in literary medical journalism.[54] Indeed, after Sacks's second book, *Awakenings* (1973), was received warmly among lay readers, his medical colleagues excoriated or simply ignored him, with medical journals refusing outright to consider his more clinical articles.[55] Yet it would be precisely this mode of writing that transgressed the boundaries of the clinical and the broader psychosocial world of his patients, an expansion of the patient's "history"—in essence, everything that conventional physicians keep off the charts of their patients—that would serve as a narrative model for Verghese and other South Asian American physician authors.

As scholars of his work (and he himself) have noted, Sacks found intellectual and narrative inspiration in the career and writings of Alexander Romanovich (A. R.) Luria, the eminent Russian neuropsychologist who helped not only to establish the field of neuropsychology but also to develop the Luria-Nebraska neuropsychological battery, a mode of evaluation to determine cognitive-behavioral impairment that is still used today. But it would be Luria's later writings in the "Romantic Science" vein that would serve as a philosophical blueprint for Sacks. For Luria, "Romantic Science" served as a necessary corrective to what he viewed as the reductionism in traditional scientific method, whose "objectivity" and dispassion were woefully inad-

equate to understanding how humans experience the world phenomenologically, to reanimate a language of ethics into scientific discourse.[56] Luria saw
anything less than a betrayal of true scientific inquiry, to observe phenomena
in their ecology, as an interdisciplinary approach whose fundamental expression would be narrative.[57] From his Soviet mentor, Sacks learned that this
holistic method requires observation of patients and their illnesses that goes
far beyond the clinical encounter, which in turn formed the basis of narrating case studies, or what Sacks would call "total biographies." In his classic
essay featuring the noted animal husbandry scholar Temple Grandin, who
is also known for her writings as an autistic person, Sacks argues for what he
elsewhere calls a "clinical ontology" or "existential neurology," both of which
gesture to the ethical or romantic dimensions of scientific observations that
insist on the specificity of how a condition or illness affects individuals: "No
two people with autism are the same; its precise form or expression is different in every case. Moreover, there may be a most intricate (and potentially
creative) interaction between the autistic traits and the other qualities of the
individual. So, while a single glance may suffice for clinical diagnosis, if we
hope to understand the autistic individual, nothing less than a total biography will do."[58]

The rest of the seventeen thousand-word essay "An Anthropologist on
Mars," from which this insight comes, has Sacks paying an extended house
call to Grandin not so much to examine her autism as to see how her autistic
phenomenology unfolds into the various dimensions of her life: dimensions
as significant as her career choice and as mundane as her awkward interactions with the departmental staff. When Sacks accompanies Grandin to
the experimental farm where she develops less cruel forms of slaughter, he
ruminates on her assertion that she is a "powerful visualizer" and considers
whether such reliance on visual thinking signals a primal lack that autistic
people suffer. "One might not understand what nonvisual thinking was like,
and one would miss the richness and ambiguity, the cultural presuppositions,
the depth, of language," he writes. "Was Temple's intense visuality a vital clue
to her autism?"[59] But when they are met at the farm with the sound of bellowing cows, Grandin conjectures that the calves and cows must have been
separated shortly before their arrival and observes one cow in particular moving frantically about the stockade. She announces, "That's one sad, unhappy,
upset cow. She wants her baby. Bellowing for it, hunting for it."[60] Here Sacks
narrates the specific illumination that Grandin's autistic sensory knowledge
might bring that his own sight, were it to remain narrowly focused on her
autism simply as clinical disorder, would likely have missed. Hers is a differential illumination, not a cognitive deficit.

"An Anthropologist on Mars" first appeared in the December 27, 1993, issue of the *New Yorker*, and all but two of the other chapters of the book to which the essay gave its name first appeared in the magazine. (The other two were published in the *New York Review of Books*.) Originally imagined in 1925 by its founders Jane Grant and Harold Ross (who would serve as its first editor until his death in 1951) as a higher-brow weekly humor magazine, the *New Yorker* by the mid-twentieth century had developed into a periodical that curated and cultivated writers of note and acclaim and was the venue through which significant political issues of the day might be addressed through long-form nonfiction writing. It was the *New Yorker* that published a serialized version of Rachael Carson's *Silent Spring* (1962) in advance of its release as a book. James Baldwin's "Letters from the Region of My Mind" (1962) brought the author's searing indictment of white liberalism's shallow understanding of race to an ostensibly educated white readership. And in 1963, Hannah Arendt covered the trial of Adolf Eichmann in Israel and, in five articles, demonstrated and popularized her "banality of evil" thesis. While it shared some elements of the emergent and coterminous "New Journalism" championed by the likes of Tom Wolfe, Norman Mailer, and Joan Didion—the use of fictional technique in nonfiction, such as dialogue, scenic construction, point of view, and personal voice—the *New Yorker* essays calibrated the subjectivities of their authors to restrain their potential egoism of which New Journalism was accused (often by *New Yorker* staff). The *New Yorker* essay thus served as an authoritative genre through which a physician such as Sacks could craft, hone, and disseminate the case history as total biography.[61]

The essay, like other forms of nonfiction, has long been considered a minor genre, but in the early twentieth century the Marxist literary critic György Lukács vigorously defended it as a form that could best synthesize what Luria and Snow identified as the problem of Western modernity: "Science affects us by its contents, art by its forms; science offers us facts and relationships between facts, but art offers us souls and destinies."[62] For Lukács, the essay form sublated the dialectic between aesthetic experience and the rational apprehension of concepts into a single immediate perception. Forty years later, around 1954, Theodor Adorno, in his aptly named "The Essay as Form," criticized Lukács's formulation as having it backward: the essay exposes the unresolvable dialectic between art and science and is a form so empty that neither art nor science can claim it, what he calls the potential "formlessness of form."[63] "The essay becomes for Adorno," explains Elena Gualtieri, "that space where a certain kind of thinking can subsist in a sort of twilight zone that is neither systematic knowledge nor artistic product susceptible to commodification."[64] What both Lukács and Adorno gesture to are the qualities of the essay that lend themselves to contemporary knowledge, which prioritize interdisciplinarity, translation, and legibility for otherwise potentially laconic dimensions of the world. The essay in the *New Yorker* served as an ideal vehicle for its readers, given the magazine's reputation to deliver what it viewed as socially relevant material to readers equally at home with consuming leisure products. "Throughout the magazine's history," Fiona Green notes, "advertisements for luxury goods have seemed at odds with its more serious air of social responsibility, the frivolous browsings of the window-shopper out of step with the magazine's 'reporters at large' in the wider world."[65] While Green argues that the *New Yorker* mitigated this "double speak" through self-irony—thus, its tendency to employ dry humor in its prose and cartoons—its more serious pieces of nonfiction in the form of the essay could give its readers the sense that there were some issues worth understanding that should not be susceptible to Adorno's fear of commodification.

The Education of Atul Gawande

Sacks would write his last major essay for the *New Yorker* in December 1999, but by this point another doctor had joined the staff and turned Sacks's eclectic portraits of people with various conditions into its own subgenre of the medical essay. In 1998, the *New Yorker* tapped Atul Gawande, then a surgical resident at Harvard, to join its staff. Gawande's first essay for the magazine thematized the very problem of contemporary health care: the fear that commodification and other dehumanizing practices threatened to overshadow the vulnerabilities wrought by illness and other forms of woundedness. Gawande's essay, "No Mistake" (which carried the tagline, "The future of medical care: Machines that act like doctors, and doctors that act like machines"), appeared in the March 30, 1998, issue. In it, Gawande argues, not unlike Gupta, for the benefits of advancements not only in medical technologies for diagnoses and treatments (the machines becoming doctors) but also in how doctors perfect various methods such as surgical procedures (the doctors becoming machines). Echoing the same line of thinking that pervades Gupta's work, he writes:

> Western medicine is dominated by a single imperative—the quest for machine-line perfection in the delivery of care. From the first day of medical training, it is clear that errors are unacceptable. Taking time to bond with patients is fine, but every X-ray must be tracked

down and every drug dose must be exactly right. . . . The keys to this perfection are routinization and repetition: survival rates after heart surgery, vascular surgery, and other operations are directly related to the number of procedures the surgeon has performed. . . . When I'm in the operating room, the highest praise I can get from my fellow surgeons is "You're a machine, Gawande."[66]

The figuration of the physician as machine, and the use of the term "machine" twice in this passage, is offset by the almost throwaway reference to "bond with patients," which is ancillary to true medical work. Gawande's essay seems self-consciously counterintuitive, given his acknowledgment toward its end of the alienation patients feel toward the kind of "disaggregated, mechanized medicine" that he seems to champion.

At the essay's end, Gawande returns to face the patient he has cast aside throughout much of the piece, in favor of computerized diagnosis and technical specificities of treatment, by arguing that the automation of the functional components of medical care could thus free up "generalist" doctors to "embrace the humanistic dimension of care. . . . Talk to their patients, for instance."[67] The last line of the essay reads like forced axiom: "Maybe machines can decide, but only doctors can heal." It is as if Gawande knows that the physician should be *somewhere* in the vicinity of his patient, as if he knows that reliance on mechanical figurations of medicine runs the extreme risk and likelihood of making machines of the those on whom these processes are performed. It is as if Gawande tries to imagine in the essay a thought experiment in which the perfunctory gesture to humanism in the clinic; the bond with patients; the commitment to talk to and, importantly, listen to patients are temporarily dispensed with, an optimization of medicine in which the objects of medical care—patients—never get to talk back. It is as if he allows himself this fantasy and then realizes that his *New Yorker* readers, perhaps his potential patients, might recoil in horror at the thought of his being their physician and then Gawande returns to proclaim that *of course* in the final instance the doctor will talk to patients and be there as their "healer." One doesn't get the sense, however, of what Gawande might actually say to his patients when talking with or to them, what bond he might establish in being a balm to them.

Perhaps wittingly, Gawande insists on the industrialization of biomedicine at the very moment that practitioners were responding to the critique of clinical coldness, the beginnings of patient-centered care discourse. Perhaps "No Mistake" also served as a means to demonstrate to this surgical resident that the crucible of experience of medical residency (especially one as fatiguing as this specialty, which leaves no person uncauterized), that this whole grand bargain—the rise of clinical specialization, the ubiquity of costly medical technology, the turn away from the bedside, and the misery that he likely saw on patients' faces—must all be worth it somehow. It's also the moment that doctors such as Ira Byock and Sherwin Nuland were writing about end-of-life care and medicine's inability to match this hard realism with its indelible drive to deploy technology to prolong patients' lives, whatever it takes, despite the cost in treasure and human suffering.[68] Throughout his time at the *New Yorker* and in his subsequent published books, some of which started as essays, Gawande would offer his reflections on minimizing medical mistakes, expound on the complexities and complications that inhere in medical care despite every best intention, and provide simple guidelines to mitigate clinical risk, all with increasing authority that might come from someone tasked with the translational science of describing medical culture to an increasingly wary public. In many ways, if nonmedical civilians were to wonder on any given day about medicine's futurity, they might easily, even naturally, turn not to someone *like* Gawande but turn to *him*, primed as we have become to turn to a desi doctor so well situated to teach us the future of medicine, which, in turn, might tell us what our own future might hold. Over the next decade, Gawande would contribute more than thirty essays of varying length to the *New Yorker* reflecting on this paradox in medicine: its insatiable need to colonize bodies in the name of health until a patient's very last breath, often performed by a machine. And throughout this time, the optimization of medical performance was always tempered by the specter that haunted all of Gawande's writing: the natural limits of human finitude.

The inability of medicine to maintain restitution as an indefinite narrative for the patients it serves came very much to the fore twelve years after Gawande published his first piece in the *New Yorker*. In the August 2, 2010, issue, an essay by Gawande titled "Letting Go" appeared; its subtitle asks the foreboding question, "What should medicine do when it can't save your life?"[69] The case that forms the heart of this piece features Sara Thomas Monopoli, who in 2007 was a thirty-four-year-old woman expecting her first child and had been informed by her obstetrician that she had lung cancer. Throughout the initial narration, Gawande suffuses Monopoli's story with phrases and images that suggest glimmers of clinical hope, such as the induced labor and birth of the child as a figure of reproductive futurity: "On Tuesday, at 8:55 P.M., Vivian Monopoli, seven pounds nine ounces, was born. She had wavy brown hair, like her mom, and she was perfectly healthy."[70] Vivian's birth enables Sara's team to put together an extensive and aggressive treatment plan for her cancer that has all the trappings of medical heroics to rescue a young, otherwise healthy white woman—Sara was not a smoker and exercised regularly, two details Gawande notes in his introduction of her—and bring her back into the world of the well. "She loved being a mother," Gawande recounts. "Between chemotherapy cycles, she began trying to get her life back."[71] But new tumors emerged, and by the end of the introductory section of the essay, when a third drug appears not to be stopping the spread of the cancer, the story has taken on a dramatic urgency: "The lung cancer had spread: from the left chest to the right, to the liver, to the lining of her abdomen, and to her spine. Time was running out."[72] The last sentence might suggest hopeful desperation, a rhetorical appeal to Monopoli's team, to Gawande himself, to the readers, to rally affectively and mobilize whatever medical technology remains available to save her. But this temporal metaphor to describe Monopoli's cancer and its metastasis is actually a misleading one, because the first sentence of the essay already frames the course of her illness. "Sara Thomas Monopoli was pregnant with her first child when her doctors knew she was going to die," Gawande writes, and in so doing he transforms the seemingly heroic and aggressive treatment, the race "against time," more into examples of medical sound and fury than anything approximating a cure.

What unfolds in this story of Monopoli and the persistence of medical treatment of an untreatable cancer is a compounded narrative calamity. Her eventual death demolishes the fiction of restitution, for sure, but the unwillingness of the medical staff to imagine anything but restitution erodes what little quality of life she would have in her few remaining months of life.[73] It is not only that "neither [Sara] nor her family was prepared [for her death]," Gawande writes. He also conjectures that the treatment may have shortened her life, as it certainly diminished her capacity to enjoy it: "She may well have lived longer without any of [the treatment]."[74] But what ultimately makes her story not just calamitous but tragic is its sheer ordinariness. What was once the salvific mechanization of medicine that thematized Gawande's first essay emerges in "No Mistake" as both a scene of horror ("This is a tragedy, replayed millions of times over") and the ethical crux that haunts and undergirds the essay, which he puts bluntly when he and his physician colleagues are certain of Monopoli's inevitable end: "What do we want Sara and her doctors to do now? Or, to put it another way, if you were the one who had metastatic cancer—or, for that matter, any similarly advanced and incurable condition—what would you want your doctors to do?"[75]

We might ask a related question of Gawande, one he may well ask himself: what should he, as our South Asian American paragon of medical authority, do in the case that he has presented to his readers? "Letting Go" serves as his preliminary foray into exploring questions of mortality; end-of-life care; what role, if any, contemporary biomedicine should play; and how well prepared physicians and other medical practitioners are in this role. Gawande would expand this reflection on death and dying in his fourth book, *Being Mortal: Medicine and What Matters in the End* (2014), in which "Letting Go" appears practically unrevised. Another chapter, "Things Fall Apart," first appeared as an essay in the *New Yorker* in 2007 under the title, "The Way We Age Now." But while we see Gawande's characteristic style of medical journalism in both essays—stitching history, policy, and practice with individual stories of patients—"Letting Go" bears a demonstrably more personal, even pained, tone, an elegiac affect that accompanies the almost radical uncertainty that rides throughout the essay.

Gawande occasionally inserts himself diegetically into his essays as a character. In "Letting Go," he appears midway through the Monopoli story when he is called in as an endocrinologist after a second cancer (of the thyroid) is discovered to determine whether a thyroidectomy is warranted. Knowing that the lung cancer will kill her long before the slower-growing thyroid cancer, Gawande recommends not operating but balks at explaining why. Unable to resist the optimism Monopoli feels about her prognosis spurred on by the aggressive treatment of her cancer, Gawande continues to monitor the thyroid cancer while the lung cancer is treated with experimental therapies and goes along with the prospect of her restoration to health. "After one of her chemotherapies seemed to shrink the thyroid cancer slightly," Gawande reflects, "I even raised with her the possibility that an experimental therapy could work against both her cancers, which was sheer fantasy."[76] In the televised adaptation of *Being Mortal*, a *Frontline* documentary sponsored by PBS that he narrates, Gawande makes this scene even more bald when he interviews Sara's husband, Rich Monopoli, long after Sara has died, and expresses his regret at raising the possibility of the therapy's efficacy because he knows "it's a complete lie." Rich smirks and retorts, half-jokingly, "You could lose your license for that." Gawande chuckles and says, "I know."[77] Monopoli's and Gawande's attempts at levity, however, belie the dread, even horror, of this scene: a physician risking malpractice by lying to a patient about her prognosis, because "discussing a fantasy was easier—less emotional, less explosive, less prone to misunderstanding—than discussing what was happening before my eyes."[78] Gawande is completely bereft of authority in this scene, lacking both the art of communicating compassionately and honestly with Sara and the medical science through which she might have made better decisions for the remainder of her days.

In her reading of Gawande's first book, *Complications* (2002), Lisa Diedrich argues that the physician author's ongoing engagement with the "fallibility, uncertainty, and mystery" that circumscribes the contemporary medical enterprise leads him to develop in his writing an "ethics of failure" or "an ethical project that emerges from what medicine doesn't yet know."[79] Diedrich sees in Gawande's attempts to improve medicine's "imperfect science" a practice of "medicine at a loss"—that is, an acknowledgment of the gap between its claims of knowledge and what lies beyond its knowing—and in this gap "to not turn away from suffering."[80] Certainly, Gawande's own actions in "Letting Go" rehearse medical failure, but his interaction with the Monopolis is a decidedly *unethical* act. "Letting Go" points not just to medicine's limit, but also to the limits of Gawande's own "ethics of failure": his lying to the Monopolis about Sara's inevitable death by failing to disclose what he already knows, and what medicine itself knows, of terminal prognoses reveals that medicine's failure may very well be an ontological one. It is for sure a structural one, as Gawande himself recognizes when caring for people with terminal illnesses. "There is almost always a long tail of possibility," Gawande writes, "however thin. What's wrong with looking for it? Nothing, it seems to me, unless it means we have failed to prepare for the outcome that's vastly more probable. The trouble is that we've built our medical system and culture around the long tail. We've created a multitrillion-dollar edifice for dispensing the medical equivalent of lottery tickets—and have only the rudiments of a system to prepare patients for the near certainty that those tickets will not win."[81] His rhetorical question—What's wrong with looking for this long tail of possibility?—actually suggests that there is much wrong in this biopolitical goal of medicine: medicine as a fantasy-industrial-complex.

The title of "Letting Go," then, evokes not simply resignation at the fact of death, that patients should let go of reproductive recovery, or that physicians need to let go of trying to save patients' lives at all costs, material, affective, and otherwise. Gawande suggests something that is perhaps unintentionally more radical: medicine may need to let go of itself in order to save itself. To this extent, the answer to the subtitle's question—"What should medicine do when it can't save your life?"—is a stark one that Gawande insinuates but can't bring himself to verbalize: nothing. To move from an ethics of failure to a pedagogy of refusal may ultimately prove to be a move too far for most, if not all, physicians, but the final scenes of Sara's tortured life before her death rehearse what this might look like. Gawande recounts Sara's last day of life: the Monopolis head to the emergency room as Sara suffers from a severe bout of pneumonia, where her primary care physician remarks, "Sara looked ghastly."[82] After the medical team is initially allowed to treat the pneumonia with antibiotics, a palliative care team is called in and immediately relieves Sara of her pained breathing after giving her a dose of morphine. Sara's family decides then to stop all treatment, and after a long night of Cheyne-Stokes breathing, a form of respiration that many dying people express, Rich tells Sara to "let go." Sara dies later that morning. Throughout this section, Gawande writes in a kind of vérité journalistic style, simply following one character to the next without fully synthesizing the scene into diagnostic outcome. Gone is the temporal urgency that Gawande narrates earlier in the essay. The scene is not even elegiac, as if taking that tone would be to imprint or impose the emotions of the physician onto these final moments of Sara's life. Gawande matches the solemnity of the tone with a very light presence, as if the prose itself needed to be breathless so as not to disturb these final moments between Sara and Rich. "At least she was spared at the very end" is Gawande's heaviest intrusion.

This coterminous lightness and attentiveness is akin to what Rita Charon metaphorizes as the cardiac work of doctoring, of which there is the systolic dimension: "diagnosing, interpreting, generating hypotheses that suggest meaning, making things happen." But "at almost the same time," Charon continues, "or alternating with this systolic work is the diastolic work—relaxing, absorbing, making room within myself for an oceanic acceptance of what the patient offers. In the diastolic position, I wait, I pay attention, I fill with the presence of the patient."[83] The diastolic "work" of medical practice, a kind of anti-work, is both Gawande's goal and his method at the essay's end, of letting go of medical action toward a form of counterintuitive passivity. While the essay broaches some "better" practices that medical personnel might deploy for end-of-life care—palliative and hospice care, clear and simple advanced health-care directives, developing best practices in engaging patients in such conversations—it ends with neither a comprehensive plan nor a call to action to develop such a plan. Instead, the narrative ends when Sara dies, Gawande's silence as diastolic witness.

There is in this silence something that turned or changed in Gawande, not quite a trauma but an experience, still, that was indelible to him as a physician and as a writer teaching his *New Yorker* readers about medicine and its cultures. Sara Monopoli suffered an untimely death—untimely in part because of her relative youth and health at the time of her cancer. But then there's also the suffering and untimeliness of the aggressive treatment that ironically robbed her of the quality of time, however short, she might have enjoyed with her husband and baby daughter. She thus comes to represent for Gawande precisely the figure that medicine should have healed but whose efforts, having the completely opposite effect, revealed—in its political economy, in its culture, in its biopolitics of the most intimate sort—something of medicine's monstrosity, as relentless as Sara's cancer itself. Medicine, Gawande realizes, to his horror, can't help but metastasize. "Letting Go" is an essay that glimpses this shadow of Gawande's profession and probes the possibility of illumination that comes from a pedagogy of refusing the medical imperative of action. "The law of the innermost form of the essay is heresy," writes Adorno in "The Essay as Form." "By transgressing the orthodoxy of thought, something becomes visible in the object which it is orthodoxy's secret purpose to keep invisible."[84] Gawande's heresy in "Letting Go" stems from his understanding that medicine can't help but try to act, to intervene, to fantasize its salvific capacities, and he, as a physician, couldn't help but fantasize with the Monopolis, against all of his medical knowledge, that experimental drugs for lung cancer might also attack her thyroid cancer. It is this traumatic kernel of memory that Gawande returns to in the essay and in the television version, which he must laugh off lest he be shattered into silence by its import, and that ultimately leads him to narrative silence and ethical passivity.

We might think of the case of Sara Monopoli as haunting Gawande's writing career henceforth. Gawande continued to contribute to the *New Yorker* after "Letting Go," even writing one essay, "Big Med," on an earlier ethos of employing systems analysis to make medicine "better." In "Big Med," Gawande wonders what medicine can learn from the multiscalar operations of none other than the Cheesecake Factory.[85] But the volume of his writing has decreased dramatically, and much of it has focused on health-care costs and the future of the Affordable Care Act, especially after the election of Donald Trump.

"Letting Go" and an earlier essay on aging formed the pillars for Gawande's fourth book, *Being Mortal: Medicine and What Matters in the End* (2014). The first five chapters describe, characteristically in a systems approach, the challenges of aging: both the physiological and the phenomenological experiences of journeying through old age toward death via illness and disability, as well as the various modes of autonomy, community, and habitation that the elderly must endure (nursing homes) or might actually enjoy (newer independent or semi-assisted-living facilities). "Letting Go," virtually unchanged from its *New Yorker* iteration, is the book's sixth chapter. Yet it retains an affective, heretical power, not only for its own story, but for its prescience for the final two chapters, which is where Gawande's book makes a decisive turn to the very personal: his father's own experience with cancer and with dying.

If Sara Monopoli's story served as an object lesson that haunts Gawande for the misery of medicine's biopolitical hold on people to the bitter end, Atmaram Gawande's experience of disease and death expresses the possibilities that emerge when the pedagogies and practices of refusal—doing less and sometimes doing nothing—are embraced. Diagnosed with cancer of the spinal cord a little more than a year before Sara Monopoli was told about her lung cancer, Atmaram, who was a practicing surgeon himself, initially takes the advice of a physician who, as Gawande recounts appreciatively, listened to his father's fears of immobility and paralysis and followed a course that doctors call "watchful waiting"—that is, simply observing by experience and testing the course of a tumor and its effects on the body. Two and a half years later, in 2009, however, Atmaram's symptoms have worsened appreciably. His limbs have begun to fail, and he and his family are worried about quadriplegia. Girded with—or, rather, chastened by—the haunting lessons of the Monopolis, however, Gawande asks his father questions not made available to Sara: his fears about his disease, his goals if his condition worsens, and when, in essence, he should be allowed to die, to let go. "These questions were among the hardest I'd asked in my life," Gawande writes, "but what we felt afterward was relief. We felt clarity."[86] Gawande pauses biopolitical medicalization for a moment of diastolic listening, which affords the entire family a new narrative that they could co-create, a narrative unavailable to the Monopolis because of the relentlessness of medical action.

Still, even with, and despite, the wishes clearly known by his family, Atmaram suffers from the fantasy of restitution in medicine. After surgery to remove the parts of the tumor that bring him the most pain gives him enormous relief, he relents to radiation therapy at the advice of specialists and Gawande himself. He not only experiences extreme side effects, but there is no reduction in his tumor. If this weren't bad enough, another oncologist recommends chemotherapy, telling him, even after relaying that the likelihood of effective tumor shrinkage hovers around 30 percent, that he "could be back on a tennis court this summer, hopefully."[87] Gawande is incredulous and apoplectic, possibly because the oncologist's suggestion mirrors how he has engaged patients such as Sara Monopoli: "She [the oncologist] was driving exactly the conversation that I myself tended to have with patients but that I didn't want to have anymore."[88] So from this point forward, Gawande serves as his father's interlocutor, advocating forcefully for his father's wishes to prioritize not suffering and experiencing extreme pain. Gawande, his mother, and his sister watch and care for Atmaram, not without difficulty and grief, in his slow and then quick decline toward death. After saying that he wishes to die in his sleep, Atmaram does just that. Gawande's final observation is of the family realizing, almost fleetingly, that his father had simply stopped breathing—or, as he ends the chapter: "We went to him. My mother took his hand. And we listened, each of us silent. No more breaths came."[89] The one, crucial thing that Gawande learns in the Monopoli case, which he narrates as a simple observation of Sara's final breath, is replicated here in describing his father's silence and listening as deliberate passivity, a mode far away from his authority as a physician.

Gawande's bearing witness to his father's self-narrative of his end; of once again becoming and dying as a person and not only, or no longer, a patient; of engaging mortality as a form of agency all signal the mode of pedagogy that South Asian American physicians are now being called on to demonstrate in the contemporary United States. Like the kind of effortless performativity that physicians are expected to show in the clinical setting, South Asian American physician writers display a command of language that overwhelms the reader in its ability to turn the complexities of biomedical science into elegant prose, in effect to rehumanize the potential clinical coldness of medical language into a language that can reach the level of the literary. In Gawande's case, the essay begets the memoir, the taking of his medical and literary erudition to its limit, only to culminate in writing the deeply intimate: Sara Monopoli to Atmaram Gawande. It is not at all coincidental, I think, that Gawande, among the most popular and critically acclaimed authors of medical science in the contemporary moment, was a Rhodes scholar. (The Rhodes Scholarship is considered among the world's most prestigious and a strong expression of Western cultural achievement.) While many Americans, seeking to optimize their health in the long shadow of biopolitical misery wrought by contemporary biomedicine, have been drawn to South Asian Americans in the form of gurus such as Deepak Chopra, whose pseudoscience is matched by their hackneyed, koan-like prose, it would take the literary acumen of Gawande—and Verghese—to suture once again the arts and science and even find the language to put medicine in its place. In perhaps an unwitting jab at Chopra, the epilogue to *Being Mortal* begins with Gawande asserting medicine's final frontier, a future that feels almost impossible but necessary all the same: "Being mortal is about the struggle to cope with the constraints of our biology, with the limits set by genes and cells and flesh and bone."[90] Sometimes, Gawande implies, medicine's place is outside the deathbed, and maybe this is okay.

Or, perhaps, we want the doctor there at our end, as long as he is South Asian American. Luther Hines, the last patient about whom Verghese writes in *My Own Country*, before he leaves Tennessee for a new position in El Paso, Texas, is, like his other patients, terminally ill from AIDS and various complications. Hines is also the most intractable and uncompliant of all of Verghese's patients, the one Verghese thought wouldn't live three days after their first encounter but who lived for two more years, with tuberculosis, candida, and other infectious miseries. He is a man full of rage and chaos. Verghese describes the moments of this final examination of Hines:

The sounds of my percussion on his body fill the room. *Thoom, thunk, thunk, thunk, tup, tup, tup.* I glance at his parents. They listened to the sound of their son as if mesmerized. Once more: *thoom, thunk, thunk, tup, tup*—even Luther seems to pause in his delirious muttering, his floccillation, to listen to the music of his body, to relax, to smile. My tools—the hammer, the flashlight, the stethoscope—are scattered on his bed. As I pick them up one by one, I realize that all I had to offer Luther was the ritual of the examination, this dance of a Western shaman.[91]

It is this final self-figuration of Verghese as the physician turned shaman that is striking, and it may provide an insight into the role that is expected of the South Asian American physician, undone by his very skill. It is the South Asian American physician at home in Western medicine and in literary erudition crossing over into the role of the medically useless shaman—Verghese's doctor as guru, as opposed to Chopra's guru as doctor.

A Part, yet Apart: Sunita Puri's Pedagogy of Medicine's Ends

Twenty-five years after Verghese transmogrified from infectious disease specialist to "Western shaman," and about a decade after Gawande painfully learned to "let go" of the algorithmic imperative of medical diagnosis and treatment that made Sara Monopoli suffer so, Sunita Puri recounted her final rotation as a fourth-year medical student assigned to the then-quixotic subspecialty of palliative care. In *That Good Night: Life and Medicine in the Eleventh Hour* (2019), her memoir chronicling her life and career as a palliative care physician, she observes Dr. McCormick counseling Donna, a woman experiencing end-stage renal failure whose medical team wants to increase her visits to dialysis. But as Donna's fatigue noticeably overwhelms her, Dr. McCormick steers the conversation toward topics that Gawande and Verghese might subsequently reflect on through their writing but, as they document, still trouble them and their South Asian American male colleagues in their actual encounters with patients. McCormick describes what will happen to Donna if she stops dialysis, then lays out a treatment plan to mitigate her pain, to ease her toward the end of her life, a "merciful way to die." "I had never seen this type of doctoring before," writes Puri. In "find[ing] purpose in a field that embraced what medicine sought to erase," that disease eradication might no longer be the only path to alleviating suffering, and perhaps not even the principal one, Puri begins a career whose principal vocation is to help all whom she encounters—patients, family members, health-care colleagues—let go as constitutive of the essence of medical practice.[92] Against the systolic impulse and drive to act and treat, Puri moves diastolically toward modes of inaction: "We all learn how to do things to patients, but not how to undo them."[93] It would take a whole career, a lifetime, for the exceptional South Asian American men to undo and unlearn the soteriological role foisted on them to stand at the bedside of the dying and do nothing, and say nothing. It is where Puri, our first published South Asian American woman physician, begins: "There is no script, no training course, that can teach you how to sit in silence, how to listen to [your dying patients]. . . . You remind yourself that it isn't your job to erase or justify all of their suffering, but rather to see it, not ignore it. To ease it when you can. And to be there as they move through it, as it passes through like clouds in the sky."[94] The limits of medicine, constituted by the finitude of human life, are Puri's ends, which compel an altogether different pedagogical imagination of clinical space and practice. Like Gawande before her, Puri was a Rhodes scholar, which surely primed them both to bring the world of biomedicine into the literary imagination of those still not yet at home in the hospital. But while Gawande began his writing career to restore to readers the human dimensions of medicine, only to realize belatedly the regime's insistence to colonize knowledge and bodies, Puri's memoir signals a shift in what constitutes South Asian American medical exceptionality. Puri's journey as a physician has her walking away from her male desi colleagues to imagine the white coat of her profession—of illness, dying, and death—not as problems but the places from which meaning, purpose, and even new stories might emerge. Just as Jhumpa Lahiri deliberately decided to give up the language of mastery for one without the guardrails of outcomes and expectation, Puri would have herself and her fellow doctors not as embodied hegemons but as co-creators of suffering. Who else might follow?

2

The Doctor, Undone

The Rise of Physician Chaplaincy

Cruelties of Competence, Epiphanies of Unlearning

The author Nora Gallagher reflects on the moment in which she "drop-ped out of the world I lived in . . . and entered another country," this other country being the land of "disease and vulnerability and death and *all that*," as a moment triggered by a single word from her doctor: "Darn." Her physician's profane shibboleth hurls Gallagher into this other "country," a geopolitical figuration of illness often used in illness memoirs, one that approximates the chaos wrought upon those given an unexpected and life-altering diagnosis. This other country, what Susan Sontag famously referred to as the "kingdom of the sick," is a land without many guides or clearly defined routes; the "all that" is Gallagher's wry way of gesturing to this chaos, what one might call a wilderness if you wanted to extend the geo-graphic metaphors. "Darn" is uttered by Dr. Marc Lowe, an ophthalmologist whom Gallagher describes as a "lean Chinese American man whose uncle is a surgeon in Beijing," and who immediately subjects her to a battery of tests at his office and then at a rheumatologist's office down the street.[1] These tests are part of "all that." Thus begins the long flight of illness and treatment for optic neuritis, as well as her struggles with her Christian faith, that forms the story of her memoir *Moonlight Sonata at the Mayo Clinic*. Dr. Lowe appears only once more in the narrative, when he urges Gallagher to visit a neuro-ophthalmologist at the University of California, Los Angeles. While Galla-gher thanks him on her acknowledgments page for his "early identification and quick response," she decidedly focuses on other doctors for enabling her to "persist," as she puts it, during treatment. Indeed, she dedicates the book to the "good doctors," as well as a physician's assistant. Dr. Lowe is not listed among this group.

I begin with Gallagher's story to highlight one way that Asian Americans occupy the contemporary landscape of narratives related to the health-care industry and the experience of illness and disability. Narratives of illness and disability, of which Gallagher's is one of so many in what G. Thomas Couser calls an illness and disability memoir boom, tell stories both of illness and medical treatment, and it is often not clear what dimension is worse for the narrator.[2] In Gallagher's telling, Dr. Lowe emerges as the observant, competent physician whose technical acumen enables "early identification and quick response," but little more than that. He doesn't help Gallagher in her existential plunge into this other country, which she calls "Oz," another figuration of Sontag's kingdom of the sick. Rather, his role is to identify her as ill and illness as a kind of existential even ontological condition, then turn her immediately into a good patient; within minutes of the diagnosis, Gallagher has an IV placed in an arm's vein as Dr. Lowe takes more pictures of her eye. The medical sociologist Arthur Frank would view this activity as an expression of "modernist medicine," in which the doctor assumes narrative authority, with technology at his disposal, while correspondingly the now newly diagnosed ill person is turned into a "patient" insofar as she allows the doctor to craft the story of her ill body.[3] Gallagher learns to speak when asked a question by the doctor. Her identity as a patient is tethered to the approval of those charged with caring for her. She is now first and foremost a patient, with all the implications of passivity embedded in the word. The fact that Dr. Lowe is Asian American is unremarkable; he is part of a medical demography that doesn't surprise: alongside the post-1965 migration of South Asian foreign medical graduates (FMGs) and their second-generation children, also medicine-bound were waves of other Asian immigrant and U.S.-born Asians who would populate the medical profession. The most recent data from the American Association of Medical Colleges counts one in five practicing physicians to be of Asian descent, with that percentage increasing as Asian American enrollment in medical schools continues to rise.[4] What is striking about Gallagher's doctor is how *unremarkable* and *unimpressive* he is, this physician who plunges her into a world of subjection and examination and interruption and contingency and who can do little more than make sure that she's "in the system" by the day's end. Yet Dr. Lowe has done nothing clinically wrong. In fact, he demonstrates nothing but medical competence, even as it is clear from Gallagher's memoir that such competence not only didn't alleviate her suffering but actually added to her misery. As Atul Gawande demonstrated in the previous chapter, under the searing conditions of his treatment of Sara Monopoli, and as Dr. Danielle Ofri has recently written about the linguistic problems that plague the contemporary physician-patient relationship, the algorithm of medical examination itself contains a brutalizing force, an interpretative violence that makes the "becoming patient" as awful as the illness itself.[5]

We see in Chapter 1 that it often takes both the long fetch of a storied medical career, punctuated by a crisis that disrupts the authority born of this same successful career—think Luther Hines for Abraham Verghese or Sara Monopoli for Gawande—that moves the exceptional South Asian American physician to reimagine his role, radically, from agent of medical heroism to mere bystander to mortality's inevitable triumph. It is a paradox out of which Sunita Puri, our South Asian American woman physician, has forged a professional career; she distills the vexations of Verghese and Gawande into a precise question, by asking medicine to reimagine its ontology when she asks toward the end of her memoir, "I wondered if, at this moment in the history of Western medicine, an important revolution could consist of both pushing the limits of nature while simultaneously accepting our patients' mortality, nature's ultimate limit. Can we do both as physicians? Can we strive to minimize the suffering inflicted by disease while also embracing more fully the truth that mortality is not a condition medicine should seek to cure?"[6] In imagining a serious and honest answer to this question, Puri seems to suggest an altogether different organization of medicine's political economy, not to mention its affective orientation—she imagines a future in which a palliative care is no longer a subspecialty but, rather, constitutive to all health care—that would make the doctor's vocation an altogether different one that might have attended to the existential crisis that Dr. Lowe was certainly ill equipped to consider with Gallagher. In Puri's estimation, physicians would be at the ready to respond to the despair that Gallagher and other ill people feel when their bodies break inexorably and wonder what it all means, a response that neither fixes nor answers but sits with the question and the brokenness as a form of interrelation.

Does it matter that Puri is a woman as she comes to this narrative realization? This chapter does not argue any form of gender essentialism, any suggestion that aligns physicians' gender with their capacity for care that goes beyond treatment algorithms. It does note, however, that the preponderance of physician memoirs written by women that intentionally take up *how to care* as doctors is also not mere coincidence. Patients encounter their physicians in the totality of their social identities (both patients and doctors), so it should not be surprising that something similar is being asked of women who write about their experiences as medical professionals. If a gendered expectation of caregiving exists that is mobilized in imagining what one's doctor can and should do, such readerly reception might correspond. This would be as unsurprising as it is annoying, as it leads us down the aforementioned cul-de-sac of essentialism. But we need not end here. We can ask what else might come of expanded and expansive thoughts of care that for sure begin from women's narration but need not end there, just as a feminist ethics of care may have started from the lived experiences of women but ideally can be generalized beyond them.[7] What Puri alludes to in her question, and the authors examined in this chapter point to in their memoirs, are the narrative possibilities born of imagining medicine not as didactic or algorithmic—getting folks "into the system"—but as moments and encounters of hermeneutic plenitude. Arriving at this disposition ultimately has less to do with gender (though again, the expectation pushes the women there sooner and more often) than with the extent to which our physicians discover a willingness to view their interactions with the ill not merely as occasions of their interpretative genius but, instead, as opportunities for interrelated, even interdependent, forms of meaning making.[8] These authors bear no special insight at the outset, mind you. Rather, what they share is a willingness to consider forms of radical unknowing, a kenosis of possibility, into which someone else must finish the story—more often than not, their patients.

This chapter doubles down on the until recent fact that the predominant Asian American narrative, as it relates to illness, has been and, for the foreseeable future, will continue to be the physician memoir. This historical, specific emergence of the Asian American medical narrative might be understood in two distinct but related ways. First, as we saw in the case of our South Asian American medical colleagues, the physician's story reinforces and distills the prevailing social narrative of Asian Americans as model minorities, a narrative far more durable and plastic than the people expected to live them. Indeed, I've argued elsewhere that the representation of Asian Americans as model minorities coincides with this ongoing passionate attachment to fantasies of indefinite health.[9] Asian American physician narratives buttress this connection, for which group is better positioned to be non-sick people than professionals who are existentially and socially produced to diagnose and cure what ails you? There are myriad reasons for why this is so. The political economy not only of the United States in the past half-century, coupled with the educational infrastructures of many developing economies in Asia, offers one piece of the story. South Korea, for example, built medical and nursing schools in the aftermath of the Korean War specifically to train young doctors and nurses for export to the United States, with curricula modeled after U.S. schools to facilitate easy licensing. This occurred around the very time that the United States transformed its immigration policy to a new mode of state selectivity, displacing national origins for employment-based preference at the very moment that demand rose for skilled health-care workers. (We see similar demand for skilled technology workers from Silicon Valley today.) Layer onto this the passing of this notion of social progress to the second generation and you can imagine how it became an easily reproducible narrative into which Asian Americans could project desire. Both the entry of highly skilled professional immigrants and the reproduction of such selective productivity in the second generation highlight the extent to which the Immigration Act of 1965, so lauded as an example of a more relaxed immigration policy compared with older versions based on national origins, still retains and even deepens the United States' commitment to what Tobin Siebers calls the "ideology of ability" at work in such policy. What was true for South Asian FMGs immediately after Hart-Celler remains de facto and de jure contemporary immigration policy, one that continues to desire the educated, the productive, the able-bodied, ready at the outset to enable the further capitalization of human resources immediately upon arrival.

But if we leave the story there, what we are left with is a fairly flat story, as unremarkable as Gallagher's Dr. Lowe. Asian American physician narratives, as we saw in Chapter 1 and extended in this one, also demonstrate the failures of medical heroism. Indeed, it is often the moment of crisis that interrupts the progressive story of medical success that reframes and catalyzes the onset of writing about their experience as doctors. In short, medical memoirs emerge from, describe, and process crises that challenge the hegemony and ideology of modernist medicine. The question that emerges from these competing agendas in Asian American medical memoirs, then, has to do with the production of identity after the crisis of faith. Indeed, one might go as far as to say that, to the extent that the Asian American's story's telos is the physician's, the memoir becomes the occasion through which the Asian American reframes and reconsiders this notion that the physician is the model minority par excellence with some circumspection, if not more full-blown ambivalence.

Memoir as Genre as Racial Form: Michelle Au

Asian American medical memoirs don't differ all that much from other American medical narratives, insofar as many of them tend to focus on that crucible of experience that is medical school and, later, residency. It is the latter that often prompts the writing: the days of exhaustion, the intense pressure, and the deep concern over failure suggest that medical education is a truly transformative and disruptive process, even as it also conveys the potential triumph of medical care over illness and death. Together, the four years of medical school and the years of residency that follow constitute a disruption and transformation of identity that physician authors feel compelled to narrate, what they have become in this regimented process. Physician memoirs are strikingly consistent in their narration, insofar as almost all of them follow more or less a linear chronology to mirror the regimented temporality of their training. In her study of memoirs about medical education, which follows more than forty physician authors' accounts between 1965 and 2010, Suzanne Poirier suggests that such redundancy attests to the deeply affective and visceral dimensions that overdetermine this experience of medical education: "Medical education is an embodied as much as an intellectual process, with every cell of one's being responding to the transformation into a physician."[10] To this reading of medical education as a biopolitical process Poirier adds: "To become comfortable as 'doctor' it is necessary for effort*ful* performance to become effort*less* performativity, with an embodiment of the behaviors and attitudes that will be recognized by both patients and peers as 'doctor.' Performance is separate, different from performativity. Becoming a physician, then, is not only an intellectual but also a corporeal process, influenced by the norms that set boundaries for what 'doctor' is."[11] This biopolitical performativity of doctoring takes place in the crucible of experience that is rarely, if ever, upbeat. It is precisely the difficulty of this struggle to become—or, rather, perform—the physician's identity that would seem to make this subgenre of the doctor's "coming of age" so compelling, the ever-present specter of failure dramatizing the stakes of clinical performance.

Very few memoirs composed by Asian American physicians foreground their racial difference from their white counterparts. Think back to our brief excursus on Oliver Sacks: rarely does he make note of his whiteness, even when he is caring for and observing patients of color, and it is only with the publication of *On the Move* (2015) that he glosses over his mostly closeted sexuality.[12] This kind of racial elision contrasts with memoirs by Black physicians, for whom the journey into the medical profession often shapes narratives of racial struggle and ultimate triumph.[13] For Asian Americans, backgrounds are mentioned lightly, if at all. Take, for instance, Michelle Au's 2011 memoir *This Won't Hurt a Bit*. A daughter of two Chinese American physicians (we never learn whether they are immigrants or U.S.-born), Au reports: "Contrary to the stereotype of Chinese parents, my parents never encouraged me to go into medicine."[14] This citation of the racial stereotype, of Chinese or Asian American parenting practices that invest heavily and heavy-handedly in raising children toward value-added professions such as medicine, signals a racial sensitivity in its disavowal of its applicability to her case. Au seems, in fact, to epitomize model minority formation as she narrates her pursuit of medicine:

> Moving past high school and through college, I got a clearer sense that becoming a doctor was not something that you simply *decided* to do, but rather something that required you to jump through certain hoops and work hard toward, and as such I had done my due diligence. I stacked my transcript with good grades in science and math, padded my resume with plenty of volunteer work, and spent six months in college in a neuroscience lab doing bench research (which I hated) because I thought that at least some effort to vivisect mice was an unspoken prerequisite for medical training. (For the record: it is not.)[15]

Au's methodical but almost effortless entry into medical school does not minimize her difference from white colleagues so much as it suggests that Asian American entry into medicine is itself a racial project with an unspecified telos. The unremarkability of her virtuoso educational attainment signals racial signage well enough. Indeed, after receiving several acceptances to medical schools, Au is at a loss at what to do: "A little overwhelmed, I figured that the first thing I should do was decide which school I wanted to attend. And then what? Just show up, I supposed, in hopes that someone would tell me what to do when I got there."[16] This rather cavalier and blasé approach will shift as Au's narrative progresses, even as her casual, tongue-in-cheek style will not.

There is one more crucial dimension that might explain why so many physicians turn to the memoir as a mode of expression, what Rita Charon calls the "divides" of health care. "Health care professionals," Charon writes, "may be knowledgeable about disease but are often ignorant of the abyss at which patients routinely stand. They have no idea, most of the time, of the depth and the hold of fear and the rage that illness brings."[17] The consequence of the divides are stark and tragic; Charon reflects that physicians (whether full-fledged or in the making) and their patients "speak different languages, hold different beliefs about the material world, operate according to different unspoken codes of conduct, and are ready to blame one another should things go badly."[18] In effect, physicians and patients become different species, and if the experience of both illness and its medicalized response is the practice through which people enter the subjectivity of patients, it is the very process of becoming the physician, medical education, that instills in people the imperious identity of the doctor. Poirier notes that in physician memoirs, "The term most used to discuss *connection* with patients is, ironically, *distance*, a word meant to connote the position in which a physician can offer both compassion and sound medical judgment."[19] Physician memoirs track these ontological divides; in many cases, strive to bridge them; and in some cases, attempt to understand the processes that create them.

In many ways, the divide between physicians and patients is ridiculously obvious. Poirier puts it bluntly: "[Physicians] confront human mortality in the flesh when, on the whole, they themselves feel in the bloom of health."[20] If people who become ill are invited, or compelled, to perform what Talcott Parsons in 1951 called the "sick role"—which exempted people from normal social and economic activities in exchange for submission to biomedical treatment—then those tasked with restoring the sick person to health should very well be healthy themselves.[21] (We'll see later that it is when physicians themselves no longer sustain able-bodied, healthy status that they gain proximity to patients in unexpected ways.) Nowhere is this divide between healthy physician and sick patient more stark than in every first-year student's experience in gross anatomy, which involves the dissection of a human cadaver. Poirier writes of gross anatomy: "Many people have called it the student's introduction to death; others have called the cadaver the medical student's first patient. The students themselves often struggle to understand their relationship to their cadaver."[22] While the stated goal of gross anatomy is for students to learn every facet of the human body as a foundation for medical-science knowledge, an informal, and perhaps more significant, pedagogical function of gross anatomy is the unlearning and learning to touch another human being's body, the cultural honing of a haptic relation between physician and patient. In her reflections as an organ transplant surgeon, Pauline Chen details her first encounter with a human body in a medicalized setting: the dissection of an old woman's body in her first-year anatomy class. Noting that some of her classmates found the experience of cutting and mutilating a human body so off-putting that they dropped out of medical school, Chen confirms that she and other students learned from their teachers the first, primary impulse in medical training: "to deny their own feeling, depersonalizing the dissection experience and objectifying their cadaver. They strip away the cadaver's humanity, and soon enough they are dissecting not another human being but 'the leg' or 'the arm.'"[23] That the first clinical haptic encounter of the proto-physician demands depersonalization and objectification serves as a crucial object lesson in what will emerge as a fundamental chasm in the doctor-patient relationship. While the doctor's training begins in an encounter with dead flesh, which, in turn, transforms patients into a different species from the one the physician inhabits, the medical narrative suggests that this relation to care, to touch, to what is called the "patient encounter" remains overdetermined by this profound suppression of emotion, which produces an affect that contravenes genuine doctor-patient encounters. Chen describes this as the equilibrium that medical students develop on their way to becoming proper physicians: a new "moral paradigm [of] detached concern, secure uncertainty, and humanistic technology."[24]

Au narrates her encounter with her cadaver with decidedly less reflection. Describing dissection as, in turn, a "rite of passage" and a "holdover from an earlier age" that suffers a "growing obsolescence," she highlights the smell of the chemical preservative that keeps the cadavers "if not exactly fresh, at least intact."[25] With barely a mention of her cadaver except for a passing reference to an exposed femur or eyeball, Au seems rather unaffected by this process of touching and dissecting a human body, opting instead to highlight absurd if humorous scenes during this course. To mitigate the smells of the cadaver, she and other students change into scrubs outside the dissection labs: "Most of us at this point had lost all modesty and didn't think much of getting changed in front of our classmates. After all, we were standing outside a giant room in which thirty dead people were lying naked on metal tables under harsh fluorescent lighting. What was the embarrassment in seeing 150 half-clad live ones?"[26] While gross anatomy is the medical student's entry into what Michel Foucault refers to as the anatomo-clinical method in *Birth of the Clinic*—"All that is *visible* is *expressible*"[27]—Au's humorous gloss on such medical pedagogy provisionally deflects the reader's attention—and her own—from what is unfolding: the systematic mutilation of human bodies for the sake of medical knowledge. What embarrassment, indeed? Subject the human body to the glare of biomedical scientific vision and you leave little to no room for the shadows of circumspection or the reflective pause of something like human mystery or interiority.

When given the chance to reflect or to deflect, Au opts for the latter. She opens her memoir with an anecdote bathed in humorous, absurdist light. As a third-year medical student, she attempts to gain a stool sample from an obese patient while a resident and a nurse hold up the man's legs. Because of the patient's size, Au struggles in what is supposed to be a simple procedure, which augments her sense of clinical inadequacy. "I follow the same fold of skin backward," Au recounts, "figuring that at some point I will hit a puckered hiatus, reach in, hit pay dirt, and end this nightmare for all of us. I move posteriorly, more, and then some more, until my hand is down against the bed. Nothing but a dead end. How could there be nothing there? Is it possible he doesn't *have* an anus?"[28] The absurd contrasts that take place here—Au's search for an anus and her fantasy of the anatomical impossibility that the patient lacks one—typifies humor's classic effectiveness, of highlighting incongruity so that the reader can "fill in" the disjunctive as a way to both reconcile an otherwise unfunny moment and reveal a breached social norm. What is, of course, unfunny is precisely what is socially non-normative: a medical student searching to place her finger in the anus of her patient must be rendered ridiculously funny to mask the aggressivity and aura of sexual violence that such a scene otherwise might suggest. What biomedicine renders as not only normal but beneficial to those who have subjected themselves to its regime is the reality that, channeling Foucault again, "The patient is only an external fact; the medical reading must take him into account only to place him in parentheses."[29] Au's readers are invited to laugh at this scene so as not to respond in an altogether different manner, such as reading in silent horror what might look to others, or in a different light, like a form of spatial colonialism over this hapless patient.

Toward Clinical Mastery and Paranoid Hermeneutics: Audrey Young

One might view Au's attempt to make light of such scenes as a parodic rewriting of the physician memoir. *This Won't Hurt a Bit* contains all the telltale signs of the standard memoir: the travails of medical school, including gross anatomy; the exhaustion and insecurity of residency; the vexed relations with coworkers, especially senior residents and attending physicians; and the struggles, and often failure, to balance one's life in the hospital with life on the outside. To the extent that parody "mocks" a genre, it highlights in this case the memoir as a self-contained and knowable form. Au is keenly aware of the idioms of this form. Just as the physician memoir, following Poirier, is designed to demonstrate the movement from effortful performance to effortless performativity of the becoming-doctor, the parodic humor reverses this process and reminds readers that the education itself becomes a kind of embodied genre. She describes subtle, almost meaningless actions early in her residency that still convey gestures with some performative import. In taking her first "history" of a psychiatric patient, for instance, Au asks to auscultate, or listen to, the patient's torso: "The stethoscope is something solid to grab on to and gives me a doctor-y thing to do."[30] Later, she reflects on the pride she felt when she and other students were given pagers in the hospital: "What could be more doctor-y than having a pager on your belt?"[31] This sense of "acting the part" or being "doctor-y" is Au's way of exposing the profound, almost innate sense of inadequacy that always lurks in the lives of medical trainees, a sense of inauthenticity of which parody is a preeminent form. Parodic humor then simultaneously masks the violence of the clinic and highlights the precarity of the medical encounter, which is far less certain than biomedical discourse would have its practitioners believe.

As the memoir progresses, humor fades and gives way to pathos as Au encounters patients who will not recover from their illnesses. Just underneath the veneer of the humorous, which Au deploys parodically to mimic the performance of medicine, is the threat of its failure, after which she is left with no more idiomatic medical knowledge. Rather, her diagnostic vision fades as she confronts those whom biomedicine can't save. The first of these patients, Jeanne, is a thirty-six-year-old woman brought into the emergency room for an ischemic stroke; after a brief period of stability, she suffers what the resident suspects is a pulmonary embolism (PE). Before this rapid decline, Jeanne asks Au whether she is going to die, to which Au retorts, "No," because she "literally cannot conceive of the alternative."[32] But the alternative arrives, as Jeanne's PE sends her to the intensive care unit. At this point, Au notices less the diagnostic details of irregular heart rhythms and observes instead the minutiae of fading hope, of loss, of anticipatory grief: "Jeanne herself has not acknowledged that I am even in the room, and she stares off at a point on the wall somewhere behind my head. But as I watch, a tear leaks out the side of one eye and tracks down to her pillow."[33] After Jeanne dies, Au tries to call Donnell, Jeanne's partner, only to hear Jeanne's voice on the answering machine. "'Hi, this is Jeanne,'" Au writes, "and you could hear the smile and energy in that voice, the contrast between that Jeanne and the Jeanne that lay in the bed in Room 8 so sharp that I winced. 'I can't answer your call right now, but leave a message, and I'll promise to call you back. God bless you, and have a great day.'"[34] Au cannot mitigate the loss of Jeanne's now ghostly presence through recorded voice, which amplifies the fact of her death, humor's transgressive capacities thoroughly holstered and replaced by elegiac sentimentality. Au pays attention to silence and absence, without commentary or interpretation; it is Jeanne's dying and death that is beyond Au's medical humor, this woman's story leaving her the affective traces of pathos that Au has worked very hard to keep out of her observational and verbal lexicon.

Where Au deploys humor to contain the multiplicities of affective experience that threaten to overwhelm the emergent physician, Audrey Young invests an overdetermined earnestness, a striving for medical perfection that borders on self-righteousness. In her first memoir, *What Patients Taught Me*, Young chronicles her clinical experiences as a medical student at the University of Washington (UW) whose WWAMI program (the acronym stands for the states served by the UW School of Medicine: Washington, Wyoming, Alaska, Montana, and Idaho) sent her and other medical students to work in rural communities throughout the Pacific Northwest and Alaska. In the preface, she writes, "Finally I recognized that the only thing to really make doctoring a human act is time spent with patients. Patients teach things that the wisest and most revered physicians cannot, and their lessons are in this book."[35] This assertion of the patient doing the pedagogical work to form the ideal physician circumscribes the narrative arc of Young's memoir and ostensibly reverses the hierarchy that typically characterizes the physician-patient relationship. Yet what remains open is what patients actually teach her.

Young's first clinical excursion takes place in the summer following her first year in medical school, in Bethel, Alaska, a remote town with a substantial Yupik Eskimo community. Like most other writers who characterize their anxieties and insecurities as they approach their initial clinical encounters with patients, Young worries about her inexperience in handling people's bodies and the messiness of their diseases and expresses an eagerness to "begin caring for patients." "I looked forward," she continues, "to speaking the language of medicine and trying to make basic treatment decisions. Above all I hoped to experience human drama and emotion as it unfolded."[36] Unknown to Young, however, a profound tension lies in this clinical education, embedded in the very passage. To "experience human drama and emotion" as it unfolds requires learning to speak "the language of medicine," a form of discursive literacy that would enable Young to perform this work as a doctor. But it is this very language of medicine that threatens to create a chasm between herself and her patients, like the differential species about which Charon writes.

An early interaction with an attending physician teaches Young that, despite her desire to "learn" from her patients, it is the language of medicine that will serve as her hermeneutic. Jane McMurtrie pulls Young aside to listen to her present a patient's history and her observations. After a thorough review of the case, McMurtrie asks Young to repeat the story "without pausing." Taken aback, Young recites the history, only to be told to do so yet again, which leaves her "flabbergasted." After this third rehearsal, McMurtrie recites the case herself, "cutting all nonessentials, and finished in thirty seconds," and implores Young to "work on your presentations."[37] From this exercise with McMurtrie, Young comes to the realization that the patient's story required the doctor's idiom:

> Telling the story was the crucial first step in taking care of a patient. A presentation explained to any doctor what had happened to a patient, what treatment to pursue, and why. If I didn't know what was wrong or what therapy to give, the presentation could be an appeal for help. I was coming to a new place now. I wasn't just observing the human condition, like a photographer making pictures of what people felt and experienced; I had begun evaluating a patient's condition and was learning to speak in an equal language with other doctors. I had become a kind of activist for the sick, telling the story with my voice.[38]

Insinuating the language of medicine to become the sick person's "activist" requires a distillation of the patient's story in the service of other physicians. "Telling the story," then, is not simply mimetic but interpretive, a re-narration that privileges the economy of the medicalized version of the patient's story, which, again, is done for the sake of other doctors' ability to hear the story.

Young improves her literacy in the language of medicine as the memoir progresses, as she exults after reporting to a pediatrician her summation of a prematurely born child's perilous condition. Feeling a "rush of relief" after the pediatrician approves of her assessment, Young writes, "Now the data were ordered and organized, we'd made contingency plans, and I felt that nothing had escaped our scrutiny."[39] By the spring of her fourth year, Young recognizes her mastery over the patient's story, the perfection of medicalizing the narratives of her patients: "By month's end I could disassemble patients' stories into the smallest discrete bits and pieces, turning the parts over in my mind and trying to solve each problem with a reasoned solution. Answers to clinical questions sometimes came spontaneously from accumulated knowledge and I finally functioned with some confidence."[40] Such epistemic totality represents, at one level, the triumph of the medical hermeneutic, the ability for the budding physician to exercise the interpretive skills to craft an authoritative understanding of patients' illness stories. What her various physician teachers instill in her, and what Young cultivates herself, is a critical disposition that seeks narrative enclosure performed by the one professionally trained to perform such interpretation, a disposition that resembles certain modes of literary criticism that wish to make singular the understanding of given texts.

The Memoir as Beside the Patient

In her study of illness narratives, Ann Jurecic takes up the broad skepticism with which cultural critics look on life writing, as either naïve expressions of ideology or manipulative projects of sentimentality that obscure broader forces shaping any form of subjective expression. In the realm of literary criticism, memoirs therefore fail "both as acts of testimony and as works of literature."[41] But what drives this dismissal of memoir, Jurecic insists, is a privileging of the critical hermeneutic that must necessarily be authoritative because it alone can see through the workings of power and ideology—the language of critique, in other words, properly telling the story of the memoir; the memoir cannot tell itself. "When the smoke clears," Jurecic writes, "from the proclamation that testimonies are produced by agentless puppets of power, no one is left standing but the critic who sees what the rest of us, caught up in sentiment, do not."[42] The language of criticism—or, rather, a certain mode of criticism that Eve Kosofsky Sedgwick refers to as "paranoid reading," a suspicious hermeneutics that require a deft critical capacity to know a text better than it knows itself—is one that, Jurecic argues, is the domain principally of affect theorists but a project that extends well into other subfields of cultural criticism, from the symptomatologies of psychoanalysis to the materialism of historicism and Marxist readings to the loosely arranged "movement" called New Formalism. In many cases, the structural imperative and incentive of the contemporary humanities place primacy in asserting the critic's ability to know more, see beyond, and understand better.

If the cultivation of a professional readerly practice by the discerning critic renders the memoir as a genre on which to cast deep skepticism, then something akin, and even more insidious, takes place as emergent physicians learn to tell the patient's story. Like their colleagues in literary criticism, these patient narratives are modes of communicability among colleagues; a patient's understanding of her medicalized narrative is secondary, at best. Only the patient's content of the story matters, as it must then find a medical form for its expression, a kind of medical formalism that is the only legitimate mode of patient storytelling. When Young discovers her ability to distill the patient's story into discrete, usable bits, she harbors not a little pride, both an intellectual and emotional realization of her coming of age as a true physician. Such is the necessary educational culture to complete the circuit of Parsons's sick patient role: if we are going to exempt the ill person from the normative expectations of work, provided that she submit herself to the observation and treatment of the professional, then what also must be placed under submission is the story of the patient's illness for medical editorial.

For her part, Young tempers this interpretive tyranny of medical reading practices as she continues to meet patients, many for whom such hermeneutic hegemony doesn't cure them of illness or alleviate their suffering but, more often than not, prolongs it. Even as she basks in her pride that she can do what her attendings insisted that she learn—to read patients with medical efficiency—she comes to realize (or, rather, remembers) that the patient's ill story exceeds medical explication of her body as text. This excess Young calls the "human": "Then the human story reasserted itself boldly and swept me to a place I recognized immediately as a place of danger and compromise, where I ought to pay close attention and tread with great care."[43] The danger and compromise, Young discovers, are the instances that lead Au to drop the parodic humor in her telling, those encounters when even the most precise medical close reading fails to produce its intention, which is to restore people to health. For both Au and Young, then, it is medicine's failure to totalize the experience that patients undergo—or, perhaps, more to the point, when its practitioners cede the medicine's territoriality to other ways of observing patients, a "great care" beyond biomedical investment—that provides a mode of *being with* (rather than doing to) patients that doesn't resort to diagnostic criticism.

Before she died in 2009, Sedgwick had developed a different reading practice from what she saw as the "staple of critical work" of the past forty years, what she calls the "beneath" and "behind" modes of criticism.[44] Later, she would call this "paranoid reading," a hermeneutics of suspicion whose telos is the "topos of depth or hiddenness, typically followed by a drama of exposure."[45] To the extent that such criticism invests most intentionally in understanding as a form of unveiling or novel discovery, we might view paranoid reading as akin to the diagnostic urge that propels physicians to do what such literary criticism feels also compelled to do: get beneath and behind the surface to reveal the truth of a patient's story, an underlying condition.[46] But Sedgwick opts instead to lean on a different preposition from those that imagine texts or bodies laid bare for others to see:

> *Beside* is an interesting preposition . . . because there's nothing very dualistic about it; a number of elements may lie alongside one another, though not an infinity of them. *Beside* permits a spacious agnosticism about several of the linear logics that enforce dualistic thinking: noncontradiction or the law of the excluded middle, cause versus effect, subject versus object. Its interest does not, however, depend on a fantasy of metonymically egalitarian or even pacific relations, as any child knows who's shared a bed with siblings. *Beside* comprises a wide

range of desiring, identifying, representing, repelling, paralleling, differentiating, rivaling, learning, twisting, mimicking, withdrawing, attracting, aggressing, warping, and other relations.[47]

The capaciousness of "beside," which employs a spatial metaphor of adjacent possibilities rather than the necessary replaceability of "beneath" or "behind," rests on a critically altered relationship between the critic and object observed. The critic regards "beside" the object not to labor in the "x-ray gaze of the paranoid impulse . . . [to see] through the skeleton of the culture," but to "assemble and confer plenitude on an object that will then have resources to offer an inchoate self."[48] Rather than the suspicious detective—or, to extend our medical figure, the trenchant diagnostician—Sedgwick offers a model of the critic as a fellow traveler.

In their own ways, Au and Young seem to get close to realizing a role of the physician beyond that of the relentlessly pedantic critic. In their memoirs, both physicians recognize the limits of developing critical mastery over the stories of their patients: for Au, her parodic descriptions of procedures and practices on patients cannot attend to the severity or solemnity of clinical experiences; for Young, instrumentalizing patients and their stories for diagnostic ends cannot obviate other dimensions of their experience for whom her medicalized reading finally cannot reach. Both Au and Young find themselves, or are rendered, silent in the face of medicine's limits and its ends, the desire for medicine to colonize the spatial, temporal, and narrative dimensions of patients that must finally give way to the impossibility of this impulse, or the horror of maintaining this fantasy: of watching people die and its prevention, whose currency is paid in patients' suffering, or watching and letting die. Such silence is a threshold, maybe even a *mise en abyme* to another kind of narrative performance of the physician heretofore unknown or unrealized, the "great care" of Young, what Au calls the "essential humanity" that physicians must maintain, inchoate selves that seem emergent but not fully realized.

Au's memoir derived in part from a long-running blog, absurdly titled *The Underwear Drawer*, while Young's began as a private journal. Neither recounts specific moments that spurred her initial writing or her decisions to procure a publisher. In Young's account, a friend urged her to keep writing because "this could become something." But it isn't a stretch to see these memoirs as a way to come up alongside or *beside* the silence that is the event horizon of the limits and ends of medical totality. In doing so, both authors run the risk of reinscribing a totalism through literary language, humorous or otherwise, that medicine, as we have seen, already strives to do. In the essay "The Other Side of Silence," Craig Irvine argues, via a reading of Emmanuel Levinas's ethics of the call of the Other, that medicine suffers from an inability to be truly "for" the Other: "Medicine's primordial imperative may be to cure the Other, to be for-the-other, but its structure and progression are naturally for-itself, representational: it is allergic to alterity—hostile to the unknown—and thus driven by the need to *identify* everything under the 'category of the medical,' from large-scale environmental structures to the most intimate structures of the body."[49] This observation is not new, but Irvine continues when he writes that literature ostensibly suffers from a similar representational impulse: "Literature, like science, *discloses* the face of the Other (which, *as Other*, is invisible) by clothing its nakedness in forms. . . . This is perhaps why physicians respond so powerfully to literature: it mirrors medicine's representational, intentional structure."[50] But literature's representational power, while similar or parallel, is not the same as medicine's, and their parallel representational structures thus offer, for Irvine, literature's paradoxical ability to augment precisely the elements that for medicine are extraneous or diagnostically useless in its reading practice. "For medicine," Irvine writes, "literature amplifies the sound of growing grass and squirrels' heartbeats, providing a keener 'vision and feeling of all ordinary human life' [borrowing from Italo Calvino]. So doing, it pierces the 'coarse emotion' of medicine, making *unusual* the 'element of tragedy' with which physicians are all too familiar. Seeming alien to medicine, literature actually mirrors medicine's alienation. For medicine, literature represents the unrepresentability of its infinite distance from the Other."[51] While Irvine risks idealizing literature's potential to undo medicine's drive toward totality, his idealism still points to epiphanic possibilities that arrive in both Au's and Young's memoirs as silence—being at a loss for words in contrast to medicine's verbosity over the bodies it interprets—an interruption in language that can then beget new forms of language that appear ostensibly alien to literature, the clinical versions of growing grass and squirrels' heartbeats of patients' stories. Such is the potential when the doctor is at a loss for words.

Physician, Know Thyself: Sandeep Jauhar

Au's and Young's observations and recounting of their patients' vulnerabilities that circumscribe their hermeneutic impulses also elicit a disclosure of the self: in encountering the Otherness of their patients, rather than subjecting them under medical totalism, the physician authors discern a language that is also not captive to biomedical imagination. Indeed, what lurks within, or beside, their performance as doctors is less the ever-present fear of performative failure than a deeper vulnerability that compels them to then seek out words not excised and editorialized for medical instrumentality. We see this quite clearly in Sandeep Jauhar's memoir of his travails in his fraught medical education and residency, *Intern: A Doctor's Initiation* (2009). Compared with his South Asian American male counterparts' renditions from Chapter 1, Jauhar's account is far more vexed: he chronicles his decision to enter medicine and his journey through the educational and clinical gantlets as roughshod and agonizing, so much so that the experience brings him close to a breaking point and even failure. And yet it is in this extreme nadir of experience, born of bodily woundedness and attendant psychic vulnerability, that will catalyze him to write, to enter a nonmedical language as a means to remain a physician. Jauhar, through his memoir and demonstrated in the narrative, develops a way to inhabit his clinical world "beside."

Jauhar's recollection of residency mirrors Au's insofar as both relay in their narratives the difficulties of doctoring wrought by a combination of fatigue brought about by cruelly long hours, insecurities born of inexperience, anxieties about performing in front of more veteran physicians, and resentment of their relative powerlessness in the medical hierarchy. And like Young, Jauhar struggles to match his critical capacities with his superiors, to learn diagnostic reading practices to demonstrate proficiency in this critical disposition. He recounts during his clinical years in medical school an encounter with a lethargic fifty-six-year-old man. Wracking his brain for an infection to explain the man's symptoms, Jauhar orders blood tests and a spinal tap, which he performs himself perfectly (he remembers with pride). No infection is discovered, but an anomalous hormone reading suggests hypothyroidism. Sure enough, the patient's mother confirms that her son has stopped taking his thyroid medication. Triumphant, Jauhar runs into the chief resident the next morning. "Let me guess," the resident responds. "Hypothyroidism." And as Jauhar stands there in disbelief, the resident tells him how he came to this diagnosis without poking needles into the man: "I tapped on his knee." Jauhar then comments that his forgetting this clinical observational practice "caused [his] patient to undergo a painful procedure he probably didn't need."[52] Later, in internship, Dr. Carmen, the attending physician, chides Jauhar when he describes an X-ray of a patient's lungs as "wet," to which Dr. Carmen responds, "You should get into the habit of calling things by their correct name. She has diffuse interstitial edema." Carmen continues, "You have to read these things systematically or you'll miss something."[53] Like Young's desire to perfect both her diagnostic reading practices and her capacity to distill her patients' bodies into discrete bits of data easily lent to medical knowledge, Jauhar's induction into practical medical science involves reading systematically and demonstrating professional argot. But as is the case of the hyperthyroidism incident in medical school, this scene with Carmen only fuels his insecurity and dread that he is simply a poor physician, lacking in his readerly skills: "In the dark room, my face burned with embarrassment. I couldn't recall ever feeling so publicly humiliated."[54]

Jauhar's memoir highlights a physician in training who is far more circumspect about medicine, more willing to see its profane dimensions than the others we have discussed thus far. Part of the difference has to do with the fact that he also narrates himself as a far less skilled and confident physician, even more insecure than Au's absurdist stories. Much of his memoir highlights second guessing his work and his fear that he is not exceptional enough to make it in his eventual specialty of cardiology. Indeed, while Au's and Young's memoirs make scant mention of their positions as Asian American women, their Asianness sublimated into the very form of their memoirs, Jauhar's status as a second-generation South Asian American is a central thematic concern throughout his narrative, and particularly in the opening chapters. While he desired to be among the tens of thousands of FMGs who immigrated to the United States after the passage of the 1965 Immigration Act, Jauhar's father was consigned to work as an adjunct plant geneticist and his mother as a lab technician. So, as is so often the case in Asian immigrant households, Jauhar's parents made of their hard work the collateral on a debt that they expected their children to pay in the form of securing work as physicians, one that Jauhar's brother Rajiv takes up enthusiastically but that Jauhar himself initially resists: "Medicine was so bourgeois! My father admonished me for being impractical. He wanted me to become a neurosurgeon—one trained at Stanford, no less. To him, that was the apogee of professional attainment. He understood well the privileges of being a doctor."[55] Medicine represents for his mother "influence, power, and wealth," but Jauhar initially resists this imperative: "But I wanted nothing to do with my parents' dream. In immigrant Indian culture, youthful rebellion is saying no to a career in medicine."[56] Jauhar's parents exhibit the telltale signs of model minority dreaming—economic mobility, cultural capital, and latent political power—and Jauhar rejects this dream in explicitly cultural terms. Part of his rehabilitation as an Asian American recognized by his parents is his turn to medicine, his racial virtue signaling. Twice in the memoir his parents beam with pride: first, when at a dinner celebrating their father's birthday, Rajiv's pager goes off; later, after Jauhar decides to pursue medicine, he graduates on the day of his parents' wedding anniversary. For Jauhar, then, being the good Asian American (son) is deeply intertwined with being a (good) doctor, an imbrication that looms over the memoir as he struggles to endure, no less thrive, in the clinical settings of the hospital spaces that several times almost do him in.

While he measures his Asian American identity by his becoming and performing as a physician, Jauhar's sense of embodiment—and, more pointedly, his self-conscious and wounded embodiment—will propel him to write about the disjunctions and contradictions that inhere in such a formation of the Asian American physician. Half a year into his internship, Jauhar's body begins to fail him, preventing him from performing the herculean tasks expected of interns and newer residents. A herniated disk sends him into severe and chronic back pain, which both ruptures his capacity to perform his role and undermines his flagging sense of his identity as a physician. "My spirit was broken after four months of toil and compromise," Jauhar writes after he decides to take a break from residency: "The pain in my neck was unrelenting; my right arm was starting to feel heavy."[57] Rita Charon writes about the creation of multiple subjectivities occasioned by the experience of illness: "Illness intensifies the routine drives to recognize the self. . . . Illness occasions the telling of two tales of self at once, one told by the 'person' of the self and the other told by the body of the self. . . . The self depends on the body for its presence, its location. . . . The body is in the copulative position between the world and self."[58] The ill body ruptures the self into multiple subjectivities, as illness interrupts the normative temporality that the self lived in before the body fell ill. So painful is his condition that he can barely tie a tie, let alone engage with patients during rounds. "My patients joked that I should see a doctor," Jauhar writes. "My colleagues were mostly reserved, politely inquiring about the injury but not paying it much attention."[59] Jauhar's injured state embodies a paradox for the physician's identity: doctors fix broken bodies; they aren't themselves broken.

But it is his woundedness and pain that enable him to move into two other identities that, perhaps ironically, enable him to get through residency. Because he is forced to take sick leave, he is prompted to write essays for the *New York Times* in which, by filtering his own experience, he highlights problems in medical training and the education of residents and students. Certainly, the preponderance of his fellow desi male physician authors, such as those from Chapter 1, generated an ethos that allowed the wounded resident Jauhar the space to share his insights, his ambivalence notwithstanding. This writerly self emerges conterminously with his brief but significant entry into the world of the wounded: his convalescence and treatment "showed me," as he puts it, "what it was like to be a patient." Noting that he attributed to his caregivers a "kind of omnipotence," Jauhar muses, "It wasn't a stretch for me to realize that perhaps this was how my patients viewed me, too."[60] Here, Jauhar is less vaunting his medical authority over patients than, perhaps, understanding the matrices of power that inhere in the doctor-patient relationship, the mutually constitutive identities that are so much the sign of contemporary health care and so fraught with probabilities of misunderstanding and despair on the part of both. It is his time and space away from his labor as a physician, idled by his injury, that gives Jauhar not only the insight but also the time and space to write, a way to renarrate his experience as a physician, to disrupt the narrative groove of the daily grind. The idleness of his disability is the precondition for the labor of writing, a form of material and intellectual labor that makes visible the asymmetries of doctors and their patients, the hierarchies of hospital culture, and the fantasies of medical heroism, a narrative that would not have been possible were Jauhar more physically robust and able-bodied.

It is, perhaps ironically, injury and his temporary idleness that ultimately save Jauhar from giving up fully on his medical career and allow him to view his struggles in residency with some kind of redemption. By the memoir's end, Jauhar has embarked on a cardiology fellowship and realized that during his residency, and despite his incapacitating injury (or, perhaps, because of the rest the injury allowed), he has become in many ways assimilated into the very medical culture that he resisted and that almost undid him utterly. "I probably ended up becoming the kind of doctor I never thought I'd be," Jauhar reflects, "impatient with alternative hypotheses, strongly wedded to the evidence-based paradigm, sometimes indifferent (hard-edged, emotionless), occasionally paternalistic. . . . I became less judgmental—of doctors, not patients (there was a time when it had been the other way around)—and more forgiving of, more faithful to, my guild."[61] This devotion to medicine parallels his commitment to a similarly redeemed model minority identity and the reward of parental acceptance via his professional advancement in medicine: "It was good to see Mom and Dad so proud. I was 'on the right track.' I had climbed 'out of the ditch.' I had fulfilled their dream for me, and though they could never know what I had been through, I embraced their pride."[62] What Jauhar had been through was the exhausting and often overwhelming struggle of his years of residency, to be sure, but this brief pause in the sentence represents also the interruption of injury that catalyzed his turn to writing and actually enabled him to become the model minority physician he had earlier rejected or feared he couldn't live up to.[63] While he is able to sublimate his suffering during residency and fulfill this Asian American medical bildungsroman, Jauhar's career as a writer, born at the nadir of his experience, also reveals the threat of the undoing of the physician if medical education is left unreflected. Writing is the effect of crisis and itself prompts the capacity to observe an experience outside of medical discourse, a necessary supplement to the very survival of medicine's authority.

The Making and Unmaking of the Physician: Pauline Chen

Pauline Chen's memoir takes a sideways approach to her Asian American identity as she chronicles her journey from medical school to her fellowship as a transplant surgeon. Prior to her description of gross anatomy dissection and the procedure's long-term effects on patient care, she references her first experience with death, at her maternal grandfather's funeral. Chen refers to him as "Agong," which is not his name but the title "grandfather" in Hokkien, and describes encountering his body in the casket as "unreal": "I was surprised by how *un*-lifelike Agong looked lying in the casket. Despite all the efforts of the mortician, the figure in the coffin simply looked like a model of Agong."[64] Coupled with her uncertainty in facing her mother's grief, Chen registers a disassociation, even a disavowal, from her Taiwanese immigrant family member in death, which will form a primary tension throughout her memoir. Agong's "unlifelike" presentation puts Chen at a profound distance from those with whom she is meant to feel intimacy. Her Taiwanese upbringing will serve as a counterpoint to her development as a figure of medical science, a bifurcation exacerbated by medicine's desire to capture all of her imagination of life, death, and embodiment. Later, when telling her own origin story, Chen recounts that her parents sent details of her birth to a famous fortuneteller in Taiwan, who narrated her story on a scroll. "At the end of the scroll," Chen recounts, "the old man wrote a few characters alluding to my own death. There are, however, no specifics: no date, no time, and not even a word about the way in which I will die."[65] The mystery of Chen's life in this Taiwanese scroll verges into Orientalist tropes, yet Chen again dispenses with its occult or even cultural power, noting that "somewhere along its journey from Taipei to that Cambridge triple-decker and to the half dozen other places my parents eventually moved, it was lost."[66] The lost scroll haunts Chen subsequently, first representing a severing of transnational ties and perhaps expectation, not unlike the lost letter in Jhumpa Lahiri's novel *The Namesake*, in which the protagonist's intended name, to be sent from Calcutta, never makes it to the family, forcing the father to name him *ex nihilo* Gogol—an American naming ceremony, if you will. But the lost scroll will also signal a loss of the mystery, even poetry, of death (and therefore, life), for what will come to replace the fortuneteller's story of Chen's, or any other person's, life will be the calculating data collection of medical storytelling.

The anecdote immediately following this description of the lost scroll involves Chen's first time pronouncing the time of death of a patient. A third-year student in her clinical coursework, she follows Bill, an intern, after he informs her of a patient's death for which they need to write a death note. Bill is tired and bored, and his matter-of-fact demeanor matches the detached manner in which he instructs Chen in how to confirm death in a patient, after which he looks at the clock. "It was 2:23 A.M.," Chen writes. "The scraggly fortune teller popped into my head. I saw him dipping his pointed brush into the inkwell and pulling small, measured strokes across the paper. 'What do you think?' Bill asked me. 'He's probably been dead for about fifteen minutes.' He paused for a moment. 'Why don't you write that the patient died at 2:08 A.M.?' The old fortune teller disappeared. Dutifully, I wrote what Bill said and then signed my name."[67] The occult appearance of Chen's fortuneteller surfaces Chen's former relationship to death—her grandfather, her future death as a Taiwanese American—only to be dashed by the brute, profane insertion of a fictional clinical time of death. Neither she nor Bill know exactly when the patient died, so the "time of death," given legal status and power via medical fiat, is little more than an educated but still arbitrary guess. This Chen knows all too well, a loss that is the result of her joining this medical family that, in turn, supplements her detachment from her Asian American one: "I had insinuated my hand into that mysterious nexus of stars and fate and destiny, and I had reduced that great passing of life into an arbitrarily calculated moment in time."[68] Complicit in this medical colonization of the body even in death by its unilateral seizure of the patient's temporality makes Chen's fortuneteller disappear: he can't travel with her because of medicine's demand for singular clockwork.

The loss of her sense of Asian American identity through her detachment from Agong, the loss of her life-and-death scroll, and her acquiescence to the imperial demand of medical temporality coincides with Chen's figuration of life in the hospital as a form of familial surrogacy. More than simply the totality of experience that physicians in training like Chen describe, the hospital as home demands affective labor even more than the intellectual and physical exertion in the clinic:

> In the process hospitals become our makeshift homes, and the attending physicians, fellow residents, and nurses become our surrogate families. Twice a year, as a resident, I gave tours of the hospital to

medical students applying for the residency program. I always said the same thing as we passed by the cafeteria or the cluttered on-call rooms shared by a half dozen residents. "This is my kitchen," I would say. "That is my bedroom." The medical students would always giggle, but in a year's time as interns they would give a new set of applicants the same tour.

Eventually, like children, we learn to embrace the values of our new family. There is, for example, a strong oral tradition in residencies. Older residents exchange stories with new initiates, passing the culture down through successive generations in the trenches of training. Like fables, these anecdotes are infused with the values of the profession. During the early years of my training, I gobbled up these tales; I was as eager to learn them as to create some common ground with other residents. They restructured my view of the hospital microcosm, and I found ways in which my own beginning clinical experiences validated their unshakable veracity.[69]

While not ostensibly a mass market, enclosed as this "surrogate family" is in the guild of the profession, there is something of Berlant's "intimate public" in this description that runs next to the familial figuration of the hospital, insofar as Berlant writes that "participants in the intimate public feel as though it expresses what is common among them, a subjective likeness that seems to emanate from their history and their ongoing attachment and actions."[70] Of course, the hospital and the business of medical education are in fact mass markets, health care accounting for almost 20 percent of the U.S. gross domestic product, except we tend to think of patients as the principal consumers, not doctors.[71] But doctors in the making must encode themselves in the social world that they make real by affectively inculcating the business of health care into the "values of the new family," as intimate as a bedroom and as inherited as the successive generations in the "trenches of training."

But Chen's medical colleagues-turned-family is also, to use Berlant's other rich phrase, cruelly optimistic. "Cruel optimism," Berlant writes, "is the condition of maintaining an attachment to a significantly problematic object. . . . [T]he fear is that the loss of the promising object/scene itself will defeat the capacity to have any hope about anything. Often this fear of loss of a scene of optimism as such is unstated and only experienced in a sudden incapacity to manage startling situations."[72] The unshakable veracity of hospital culture to which she so attaches herself binds Chen to an allegiance to the medical regime that, over time, will turn doctoring from a privileged guild that brokers care for sick people into an alienating cult that disavows patients as resembling anything that might have the characteristics of humanity that physicians have cultivated for themselves. Like the argot that binds academic disciplines and holds lay readers at a distance, the medical profession's demand for familial allegiance will make for its Asian American physicians a culture that produces both fear of the loss of its object and the consequence of holding on to it: fear that to lose one's commitment to the tradition so carefully cultivated would be to lose one's identity after the transnational, immigrant one has been cut loose; consequence that to embrace this culture with unqualified credulity threatens an outcome far worse than the loss of identity.

This worse outcome is the cruelty unleashed toward her patients, the result of an insistence on medical optimism and its fantasy of heroism. In Chen's case, this relentless desire to uphold her faith in medicine compels her to avoid those for whom medicine can no longer stave off death's inevitability. A colleague, Kay, a receptionist in the operating room in the hospital in which Chen works during her residency, develops cancer in her liver. Chen finds herself unable to call Kay even as her cancer develops into an incurable condition. Weeks go by before Chen forces herself to call Kay just a week before she dies. Kay's son sends Chen a card and a copy of the program of the memorial service; Chen's response is to shove it all away: "I wanted to cry, but instead stashed the letter into a far corner of my desk drawer."[73] Later, during her fellowship, Chen is confronted by a stalwart nurse who asks her to pay special attention to Bobby, the nurse's former patient who is now in Chen's service for liver cancer. After a brief tumorless post-operation period, the cancer returns, and Lou, the nurse, pleads with Chen to visit Bobby and talk to his wife about palliative care, but Chen does not. When Bobby dies, Lou chastises Chen: "He was dying Pauline. He had cancer everywhere, and they still poked him and prodded him and thumped on his chest when he coded. They did the full-court press. . . . That is how Bobby died."[74]

Chen writes that her avoidance of the dying had to do in large part with how much the reality of mortality interrupted the routines she had established to nurture her optimism in medicine's salvific capacities. Her refusal to engage is indeed medicine's hail: to do otherwise, to respond to her patients in a manner that shares their suffering, would mean to reimagine herself once again as like them, which would mean acknowledging the physician's own precarious and fragile relation to mortality. Chen describes the deep and underlying tension that she faces as a forced choice between sympathy and science:

I . . . struggle to reconcile what medicine has taught me so well with the very reasons that drew me to it in the first place. I want to cry for those in whose bellies I find disseminated tumors, but cannot for fear of being unable to see clearly enough to sew them closed. I want to sit and linger with my patients, but know that such inefficiency would never work in the clinical world. I want to be able to sooth my patients' suffering without the burden of knowing the inexorable future course of their diseases.[75]

Cruel optimism in medicine begets startling incapacity. Each time Chen yearns to reach out to her patients, there is the "but" of medicine's refusal to break the narrative of its own heroism, which death always punctures.

So most of the time, when given this stark, forced choice, the tendency is to opt for efficiency and escape. Chen chronicles several tactics that she and other physicians use to facilitate the interrupted lives of the ill, to prevent the ill from verbalizing and narrating their experiences of illness. Akin to the fourteen seconds it takes for a doctor to cut short a patient telling her story of embodiment are strategies of escape and avoidance that Chen describes in terrible detail: "Whenever I was trapped in some patient's room, I could feel the next clinical task pushing at me. . . . Halfway through a sentence, I would begin to edge toward the patient's door, impelled to start moving again lest I become permanently anchored to the room."[76] Worse yet, she begins to "turf" her patients: "to send difficult, time-consuming problems to someone else," a well-worn practice employed ostensibly for medical reasons but more often than not to avoid responsibility for outcomes and inevitabilities. "Turfing seemed like the ideal remedy," Chen continues. "It was ingenuous and completely subconscious. I did not have to lie, and I did not have to divulge the truth. I did not have to see the smiles drop nor be the one to put the pin to my patients' enormous bubble of hope. In one circuitous loop of thought, I could eliminate the problem from my own vista."[77] As a culturally sanctioned procedure of avoidance, turfing is the cruel prescription for medicine's optimism. All of these "creative" ways of sidestepping, avoiding, obfuscating, and qualifying are designed, as she puts it, to displace the overarching fear that she might have to "linger in the shoes of the dying."[78] Such fear of identifying with rather than turfing those whom medicine cannot save is the deep cost to the intimate public of the surrogate family that Chen has joined. Tellingly, after Bobby dies, Chen recalls a Taiwanese ghost story, a spectral reminder of the family she left behind to join the medical one: "The old-time Taiwanese believed that certain souls haunt the world, searching for the mollification for untimely or dishonorable deaths. These *wan ong kuei*, 'wronged spirits,' are destined to wander among humans for eternity. Without any justification for his manner of death, Bobby became a *wan ong kuei* of my mind."[79]

Though she lets the fortuneteller go in favor of the clinical clock, Chen cannot fully expurgate that which exceeds the biomedical. The occult serves as the palimpsest to ill experience.

But just as Chen the doctor can be made through the imperative to adopt medicine as her family, her cruelly optimistic intimate public, so might the doctor be undone through her clinical encounters, moments that push her toward a vocation of the physician with an altogether different disposition. Three moments in particular nudge Chen to recalibrate her understanding of the role physicians should play when engaging with the ill, whether they are her patients or not. The first involves an attending surgeon whom Chen calls at home as a patient in their service, dying from metastatic liver cancer, starts to experience untreatable heart failure. Describing how she—and everyone else on staff up to that point—handles those on the brink of death, Chen writes deliberately in the passive voice, as if to highlight that the claim for patient privacy serves as a ruse to avoid engagement and, ultimately, responsibility for the dying and the grieving: "When a patient is dying in the intensive care unit, the protocol is always the same. Door or curtains are closed around the patient and family, the nurse turns off the monitors so the family does not have to hear the cardiac monitor go flatline, and physicians scatter in order to give the family some privacy."[80] This image of scattering physicians belies the privacy cover, revealing instead not only the fear, but, more important, the existential dread that being present at death brings: to face death is to be present at the failure of medicine's heroic story. Only after the family members had left the room would Chen enter and do her clinical task: "There, alone with the deceased, I pronounced the patient officially dead in three steps and filled out the requisite paperwork."[81] Note the detached adjective turned noun, as if to mimic the bureaucratic dimension of death's reckoning as mere paperwork, to mask the inability to attend to the solemnity of the moment.[82]

The attending surgeon in this case, however, does not scatter and does not neutralize the bare emotion with detachment. Contravening every experience Chen has witnessed or engaged in, the attending leads the dying man's wife into the room and draws the curtain around the three of them together. Chen wonders what to make of this break in protocol. "I peeked in," she writes. "Inside the woman was still sobbing, but she was standing with her hand in her husband's. The surgeon stood next to her and whispered something; the woman nodded and her sobs subsided. Her shoulders relaxed and her breathing became more regular. The surgeon whispered again, pointing to the monitors and to the patient's chest and then gently putting hand on the patient's arm."[83] The surgeon stays with the woman and her dying husband for a full thirty minutes; all the while, Chen hovers outside the room. She conjectures that the attending surgeon has explained to the grieving woman "how life leaves the body" and about the "final comfort of her presence," but for Chen the transformative teachable moment is for her: "I never told [the attending] that it was as if a shade had lifted ever so slightly, letting in the first rays of light, and that from that moment on, I would believe that I could do something more than cure."[84] The "more than" of which Chen writes is actually a "less than," a conscious decision on the attending's part—and, later, Chen's—to remain present with the dying, the grieving, the suffering, even in the face of medicine's inability to cure, restore, or keep alive. While the attending presumably maintains some clinical dimension in these final moments with his patient and his wife—at least, Chen speculates so—his explanatory capacity is secondary to the primary task of presence, gently asserted by a whisper, a touch, the willingness to linger, a refusal to turf. Why this scene compels Chen so much is precisely its paradox: it takes the most powerful figure of the medical hierarchy, the attending surgeon, to do the least interventionist medicine, the simple act of observation and presence, to teach Chen the "more than" of doctoring—to do as little as possible but also to remain, to stay *beside.*

While her observation of the attending surgeon allows her to glimpse an alternative role a physician might play in attending to suffering, Chen's second encounter shows her the relationality that physicians share with patients that exceeds the prescribed roles they are socialized to perform. This time the "patient" is a member of Chen's family. Aunt Grace, part of her life "from the beginning"—and, like Chen's parents, an immigrant—is slowly but inexorably dying of renal failure. Prior to describing Aunt Grace's disease and its progression, Chen notes that "doctors—like writers, artists, and spies— are professional people-watchers," a vocation of observation that is "part art, part science."[85] While commenting that the "art" portion approximates a mystical "clairvoyance," Chen decidedly foregrounds the labor of scientific observation, which she describes using a term from literary criticism: "We dismantle people as art experts deconstruct paintings. . . . Deconstruction becomes our professional tool of understanding, and we rely on it to absorb increasingly complicated clinical problems."[86] Insofar as deconstruction in the critical tradition signifies a reading practice committed to destabilizing the axiomatic and the authoritative by revealing irreducible complexities of a text, Chen's enthusiasm for deconstructing the texts of patients—or patients as texts—makes the diagnostic lens demonstrably formalist, disdainful of any kind of affect save for the physician's pleasure in discovery: "It was mentally satisfying, like taking a box of jumbled puzzle pieces, organizing them, then arranging them into a perfect picture. . . . I saw people in the grocery store or at restaurants, and my eyes would fixate on the loping gait, the barrel chest, or the finely wrinkled skin. *Stroke, emphysema, bigtime smoker,* I would think. It was strangely thrilling, the way X-ray vision might be."[87] The pleasure of diagnostic play belies the reductiveness of Chen's gaze, her professional people watching singularly trained in a reading practice of exposure, a reinforcement of and delight in the hermeneutics of suspicion.

But Aunt Grace and her ailing body stop Chen cold. While asking for medical advice regarding blood vessel grafts to improve her hemodialysis, Aunt Grace has Chen examine her, and Chen deftly provides her deconstructive analysis of her aunt. But instead of pleasure, the reading leaves Chen with a physical pressure in her head and a realization of the horrific limits of calculating deconstruction—what she calls "a prelude to a much more intense wave of grief": "The skill that had once simplified my life now left me very much alone, and the profession that had once promised the power of cure now made me feel utterly helpless."[88] If the imperial gaze of medicine renders ill people into a different species called patients, alienating them from still able-bodied humans, then the tragic and ironic epiphany here is a mirror alienation on the part of the doctor. So invested was Chen in cultivating and luxuriating in her ability to know the human body with critical rigor that it has left her alone in her grief. Her diagnostic skill leaves her no solace when examining her aunt; instead, deconstruction alienates her from her very family member. And this occurs despite the fact that Aunt Grace had told Chen throughout her adolescence and into her medical training that her listening skills and her being with people in their suffering would make her a fine doctor, the "art" dimension that Chen so quickly dispensed and dismissed in her zeal to attain the "science" of deconstructive mastery.

In her dying convalescence, Aunt Grace returns Chen to her family and to relationality. Chen asks Aunt Grace whether she's willing to be part of an article on organ donation, and Aunt Grace consents on one condition: that Chen include the stories of her husband and adult child, who had been providing progressively intense and round-the-clock care for a decade and as she approached her end. "My story is also about them," Aunt Grace insists. From this, Chen describes the last moments of Aunt Grace's life, with her family (including Chen) surrounding her: "She had become progressively more peaceful, and in the end they sat there, simply being with her, as they had always done."[89] In stark contrast to the unlifelike composure of her grandfather's body at his funeral and the often violent ways that patients die as they are subjected to "heroic" medical measures, and even differentiated from the hospital death to which she saw the attending surgeon bear witness, Aunt

Grace's death highlights deep relationality and intersubjectivity, her dying linked inextricably to the livelihood of Chen's uncle and cousin, a familial solidarity into which Chen herself is once again brought back.

What finally breaks the cruel embrace of medicine's episteme for Chen, our consummate model minority surgeon, is a haunting moment during which she confronts the closest thing to the materiality of her own body outside of her body. While the attending surgeon showed her how to remain with patients in their final moment, and her aunt, uncle, and cousin demonstrated deep relationality born of death, her encounter with a vision of her own finitude fully undoes her identity as a physician and returns her to the precarity of bare life, which, in this case, is also Asian American. In one of the final scenes of her memoir, Chen is sent to harvest organs from a woman fatally injured in an automobile accident. Although the woman is brain dead, her body remains resuscitated for organ transplant. Like Chen, the woman is thirty-five at the time of the accident and Asian American. Chen describes the moment she begins the process of entering this woman's body surgically:

> As I moved my arm to begin the incision, the sterile drape covering her right breast fell away slightly. I pulled it up again to cover all except the area of incision but noticed the undulations of each rib to the left of her breast and the very gentle fall of the breast tissue to her side. Her nipple and areola peeked through; they had a coloring and shape that I had only ever seen on one other person: myself. In fact, the very shape of her breast, the thinness of her chest, and the texture of her skin reminded me of my own upper body. It was as if I were standing naked after a shower, looking in a mirror.[90]

Without resorting to intensive psychoanalytic reading, it is not a stretch to see in Chen's mirror relation to this woman a deep investment in her proximal identity in terms of race, age, gender, and even sexuality. Chen's obsession with the woman's breast suggests an almost erotic connection to this woman. At this realization, Chen relates that she is temporarily unable to continue, stopped cold in her tracks by the thought of her cutting into her very self, a threat of violence to this woman's body that becomes a threat to her own. She continues,

> For a moment I saw a reflection of my own life and I felt as if I were pulling apart my own flesh. As we snipped away at the organ attachments, preparing to take her liver, pancreas, and kidneys, I wanted to ignore the aliveness of her body, to realize that she was in fact only

a cadaveric reflection of myself. But then I could not bear to think of herself—myself—as dead and would once again think in my confused, sleep-deprived state of her as alive. The drape across her chest continued to slip, and I would have to see her breast yet again and then cover it.[91]

Chen has difficulty "keeping [her] eyes" off the woman's skin, which so closely resembles hers, a pull of visual attraction that threatens her complete loss of medical proficiency. She then recalls that this procedure on this Asian American woman sends her not only into an "unspeakable, unbearable grief," but also into the precipitating moment that compels her to write stories about encountering the dying in her medical practice.

I would suggest that this moment, this encounter, is not simply a kind of mirror-image moment; the moment of an Other reflecting back to a self. It is also a moment of deep intersubjectivity, in which a healthy practitioner and an ill (in this case, dead) patient are not separated by worlds or species but are, instead, brought together in a kind of shared materiality. This kind of materiality is one in which life and death are not different biological states, qualitatively different clinical capacities, and not simply markers of objective time (e.g., "time of death"). Nor is this a materiality in which health and illness are separable. Rather, it is a moment of deep, visceral reality of death in life, of health as either a temporary waystation to the village of the sick or a fiction that only temporarily holds at bay the larger normative experience of illness. It is the shared materiality of Asian Americanness that binds the living and the dead together, which in this moment can only be felt but not expressed but gives rise to a wholly different kind of expression.

The Physician Author as Chaplain

Chen's turn to writing reiterates, even exacerbates to the point of weeping, "both the unresolved grief and a deep sense of shame . . . [for] what [she] had become" in her possessive investment in medical identity.[92] Yet it also enables her to end her story with a subjunctive hope for her future self as a physician. After helping a patient and his family toward hospice and a gentle death filled with family and with minimal medical intervention, she reflects: "I had caught a glimpse of the doctor I *could* become."[93] In her epilogue, Chen describes her role as a physician chaplain with her college mentor as one of companionship, the "honor of worrying" for another, in the future perfect: "And *when* we are finally capable of that, we *will have become* true healers."[94] While the subjunctive highlights the gap between what is "had become" and what she "could become" as a syntactical expression of hope, the concluding future perfect sentence speaks to an imperative for physicians to bridge the gap. This task of becoming "true healers" must happen; the physician must give up the fantasy of indefinite futurity in medicine to save it from its cruelly optimistic fantasy.

What might it mean for health-care practitioners—especially, but not exclusively, physicians—to see their identity, their vocation, their agency partly, if not primarily, as witness bearers to these narratives, so that, as Charon puts it, such intersubjectivity enables doctors "to not just feel on a patient's behalf but to commit acts of particularized and efficacious recognition that lead beyond empathy to the chance to restore power or control to those who have suffered?"[95] This, of course, is the role consigned to that most "useless" of figures in the hospital—the chaplain—insofar as the chaplain has no professional training at all to cure the patient's illness or palliate the patient's pain with narcotics. What the chaplain has in her toolkit are her senses and her embodied presence at the bedside, nothing else; she charts not disease and treatment algorithms but the growing grass and squirrel's heartbeats of the person lying right there. Chen's memoir points to this as a necessary role and responsibility, of the Asian American physician undone enough to make room for the chaplain to emerge alongside, bearing witness to the work of the physician, of the physician as witness to the reality of suffering. Imagining the physician as engaging in the work of chaplaincy might have us think through social hierarchies and other forms of sociality in the health-care profession, and even the very architecture of the hospital room and the hospital as such. Certainly, a reordering of social relationships, and of relationality to illness and ill bodies, to incorporate this materiality demands a reassessment of what actually takes place in the clinical encounter, whether it is principally a (healthy) professional identifying, diagnosing, and prescribing a bodily geography of illness that cannot know itself or this encounter is of one wounded body coming to the care and aid of another. It may involve a wholly different set of questions for the first-year medical student slipping on her first white coat; her disposition to the cadaver before making her first incision in gross anatomy class; her reading practice before she steps into the clinic for the first time; and how she might assess what she has heard. What new forms of sociality might emerge in which the stories of the ill, the stories that emanate from hospital rooms, are ones that physicians learn to come up *beside*?

3

Styles of
Asian American Illness

Paul Kalanithi: Model of Declension

By most accounts, Paul Kalanithi could have, possibly even should have, written a memoir that would have nicely fit in Chapter 1 of this book. Instead, he lies in this one. "You can't ever reach perfection," writes Paul Kalanithi in his bestselling memoir *When Breath Becomes Air*, "but you can believe in an asymptote toward which you are ceaselessly striving."[1] This sentence concludes the first half of his narrative, titled "In Perfect Health I Begin," a wry reference to the opening lines of "Song of Myself" by Walt Whitman, who wrote his iconic, form-shattering poem at thirty-seven. By the time part one ends, Kalanithi is not unlike his elder South Asian American physician statesman: having just completed a demanding and difficult residency in neurosurgery at Stanford, he embodies and expresses a faith in his specialization and, more broadly, the medical enterprise for which he feels the responsibility of the agency of the doctor in the lives of his patients: "The pain of failure had led me to understand that technical excellence was a moral requirement. Good intentions were not enough, not when so much depended on my skills, when the difference between tragedy and triumph was defined by one or two millimeters."[2] Like Abraham Verghese and Atul Gawande, Kalanithi seems to have a clear, if well-worn, path. As has been the case for our model minority physicians of the previous two chapters, medicine serves as the idealized calculus through which Asian American identities are not simply realized but recognized as authoritative, for themselves and, presumably, for a reading public who might someday be their patients. The ceaseless striving, then, in the final sentence of "In Perfect Health I Begin" ostensibly gestures to an idealized ethic of the cultured Asian American physician-writer whose drive toward perfectibility would have Kalanithi serve as yet another highly sought South Asian American medical guru of Chapter 1 to whom Americans have grown quite attached.

But this is not principally why *When Breath Becomes Air* captured the imagination of readers when it came out in 2016. By the time Random House published the memoir, Kalanithi had been dead for about nine months: the Whitman reference of part one takes on an elegiac hue, as Kalanithi died at thirty-seven—the same age as Whitman when he wrote these lines of poetry—for which part two of the memoir completes the poet's couplet: "Cease Not till Death." The ceaseless striving that seemed to fuel and satisfy Kalanithi at what he calls the "pinnacle of residency" abruptly ends, for "Cease Not till Death" opens with him and his wife, Lucy, crying as they look over the results of computed tomography (CT) scans that reveal metastatic cancer in several of his organs, a disease that will end his life by the book's end. (Paul died before completing his memoir; Lucy compiled and edited his drafts and wrote an epilogue.) Kalanithi organizes his memoir to mirror his utter transformation, from the quintessential Asian American doctor now to a terrified and uncertain person with an illness: "One chapter of my life seemed to have ended; perhaps the whole book was closing."[3] This second chapter tells the story of his book closing, but before it does, it's worth pausing to dwell on the end of the former "chapter" of Kalanithi's life. "In the beginning is an interruption," writes Arthur Frank. "Disease interrupts a life, and illness then means living with perpetual interruption."[4] The life interrupted by illness is the life undergirded by the narrative of restitution, which, resonant with the discourse of perfectibility that Kalanithi references, medicine guarantees for those willing to submit to its authority, a narrative that pivots on this axiom: "Yesterday I was healthy, today I'm sick, but tomorrow I'll be healthy again."[5] Stage IV lung cancer explodes the restitution narrative for Kalanithi and interrupts everything to which he has hitched his fortunes. And it is a perpetual interruption, a narrative wreckage. "Severe illness wasn't life-altering," he laments, "it was life-shattering. It felt less like an epiphany—a piercing burst of light, illuminating What Really Matters—and more like someone had just firebombed the path forward."[6] Illness as interruption is not always a simple pause; sometimes it is existential violence, a differential ontology by way of life shattering. Illness betrays Kalanithi's desire, his striving, his asymptotic relation to perfection now careening into an altogether different path.

When Breath Becomes Air spent sixty-eight weeks on the *New York Times* nonfiction best-seller list; Kalanithi's memoir has been translated into more than thirty languages.[7] While it isn't uncommon for highly regarded illness narratives to win both critical and popular praise, there was in the critical appraisal of Kalanithi's book a level of pathos that seems to astonish even his reviewers in their emotional reaction to the story of a dying physician, whose proof of death was their reading his memoir. "Only memory and words—in his case, those in this very book—'have a longevity I do not,'" writes Nora Krug for the *Washington Post*. "Read them and, yes, weep."[8] Henry Marsh reflects in the *Guardian*, "It is disturbing, at first, to read an autobiographical book in which the author knows he is dying and you know that he will be dead by the end of it. . . . The fact that I use the present tense in writing about him shows that the book has taken on a life of its own, as Kalanithi clearly hoped it would."[9] One might argue, and if you did you'd probably be right, that any story of death and dying of a relatively young person might be at once disturbing and so moving that one weeps. But just as the Asian American physician has served as the primary figure through which American readers and Asian Americans themselves have negotiated the perilous land of woundedness and finitude, so the story of a South Asian American doctor dying before our very eyes astounds because Kalanithi was both: he was a doctor and an Asian American, and neither doctors nor Asian Americans are supposed to die. In our era of biomedical hegemony, physicians live and must live indefinitely to keep us alive, and in late U.S. capitalism, Asian Americans secure the guarantee of economic mobility and biopolitical flourishing to maintain the social fiction that such mobility is possible. And yet here Kalanithi's body lies, revealing to us, like a revelation, that model minorities and neurosurgeons also die sometimes at the age when they are supposed to be in perfect health.

The Asian American Illness Memoir Boom

The reception of *When Breath Becomes Air*, which continued for years to take on this breathless astonishment, speaks to an important counterfactual in the memoir boom and the related subgenres of physician memoir and illness memoir (what some call autopathography).[10] As we have seen, Asian Americans have very willingly participated in building the prestige and popularity of the physician memoir, and, as Pauline Chen, Verghese, and Gawande (and Kalanithi) demonstrate, have been quite successful at it. There is certainly no shortage of memoirs written by Americans who feel moved to share their experiences of illness, injury, and disability, as G. Thomas Couser, Ann Jurecic, and Lisa Diedrich have all demonstrated in their critical surveys of this genre. Asian Americans have been writing about illness for quite some time, but not from the vantage of being ill. Rather, Asian Americans write about illness and about treating illness, as physicians. But draw a Venn diagram of these two modes of life writing—the physician writing his story; the ill or former patient composing hers—and you'll be hard pressed to find an Asian American in the overlap. This sentence that you just read I first wrote in 2014; it would have been followed by my mentioning fewer than a handful of memoirs written by Asian Americans about their experiences with illness. I would have mentioned 2011 as the year a piece of life writing by an Asian American was published for the first time: Fred Ho's *Diary of a Radical Cancer Warrior*, by Skyhorse Publishing.[11] I would then have cited Brandy Liên Worrall's 2014 self-published memoir *What Doesn't Kill Us*, her story about her struggles with breast cancer.[12] And then I would have written, "That's it," and spent the better part of this chapter reflecting on the reasons for the dearth of such writing about illness by Asian Americans.

But then something broke in the second half of this decade. The year 2016 saw the release of Kalanithi's viral memoir, as well as the publication of Padma Lakshmi's *Love, Loss, and What We Ate* by Ecco (an imprint of HarperCollins), which featured her struggles with endometriosis, though secondary to the primary themes of her failed marriage with Salman Rushdie, her careers in modeling and food reality television, and her relationship with her mother and her child.[13] In 2017, Christine Hyung-Oak Lee published her memoir *Tell Me Everything You Don't Remember: The Stroke That Changed My Life* with Ecco, the first time in U.S. history that a major trade press published a work of nonfiction by an Asian American whose narrative was primarily occupied by illness.[14] And you read at the start of this book about another best-selling memoir by Julie Yip-Williams, published posthumously, on February 5, 2019, by Random House. That same day, Esmé Weijun Wang's *The Collected Schizophrenias* was published by Graywolf.[15] It was as if, in an instant, scales fell from the eyes of U.S. publishers and readers alike: if as a collective, Americans demanded of their Asian American colleagues lives of exceptional mobility and affirmation of the U.S. cultural project, then perhaps in this surge of readerly purchase in Asian Americans getting sick and dying before their eyes, Asian America could also provide a pedagogy to optimize this narrative of inevitable declension. Asian Americans, can you teach us how to die well?

There still remains skewed written representation—an explosion of cancer memoirs, a smaller but significant flourishing of Asian American physician memoir, and a relative dearth of Asian American illness memoir, to be sure. Such asymmetry can be read in part as a sociological effect of model minority discourse. I've argued elsewhere that the representation of Asian Americans as model minorities coincides with this ongoing passionate attachment to fantasies of indefinite health.[16] Thus, we see the visible genre of Asian American physician narratives, the ostensibly non-sick professional existentially and socially produced to diagnose and cure ill and ailing America. The sociology of model minority fantasy, the success frame, has a deep somatic corollary: filial children, exceptional students, also require honed, disciplined, healthy bodies. Medical narratives represent the culmination of such collective labor, which is why this book required attention to so many physician memoirs. Conversely, to write the story of one's illness—in effect, to narrate how the body fails to be productive, fails to convert health into some kind of accumulation and mobility—punctures the figure of the Asian American as a model of social flourishing. Insofar as illness interrupts the inexorability and inevitability of the social productive body, it also has the capacity to undo the very relations of power, say, within the family, that are necessary to reproduce such model minorities into figures that may as yet be beyond literary imagination.

This genre of writing by Asian Americans, the illness memoir, is still perilously and precariously new; it remains to be seen whether it can thwart the social power of the model minority narrative and the success frame that governs Asian Americans' (and others') desire to live into it. It is, of course, true that since the publication of Betty Rollin's best-selling chronicle of her breast cancer and double mastectomy, *First, You Cry* (1976), there has been no shortage of illness narratives available from which an Asian American might model to fashion hers; the vast majority of these books are written by white authors, with a few by Black and Latinx authors as alternatives. The until recent dearth of Asian American illness memoirs once might have given rise to a peculiar anxiety—less an anxiety of influence that might characterize someone writing one's ill story in the shadow of Oliver Sacks or Audre Lorde than an anxiety of irrelevance, for who would want to read a story of a sick Asian American when the only Asian American story consistently valorized and rewarded is the model minority one?[17] Who, indeed? That Kalanithi and Yip-Williams are now oft-cited, if not household, names when recalling the illness memoir genre evidences a relatively new structure of feeling in watching model minorities die. The perforce challenge for the Asian American person trying to craft a narrative from the body that can't do what it is supposed to do—to labor to extract capital from herself and her network—rests on her living on the precipice of social unfitness and illegibility and wondering whether the success frame meshes at all with the bodily realism. It is for this reason that, as I wrote in the introduction, Julie Yip-Williams is often at pains to redeem her terminal cancer in terms of affect and futurity—the former for her in discovering wonder and awe while still alive, and the latter in passing on to her children the remains of her words. Revaluing their bodies from the stigma of unproductivity into something else requires a cultivation of narrative from which Asian America has had until very recently no sui generis resources, even fewer ways of imagining illness and death as vehicles to reaffirm the success frame. To signify illness differently, a pivot away from this insistence and imperative of productive redemption, would thus gesture to a perilous and—at least for me, maybe for you?—utopian, differential ontology.

Illness as Style: Anatole Broyard

Every writer of illness must develop something akin to an iconoclasm of style. Let's turn to two non–Asian Americans not to determine axiomatic narrative as much as to highlight how individual illness narratives can and really should be, even as ideally such stories aren't individualistic. Perhaps no writer made style his dying life's work than Anatole Broyard, the famed (or infamous, for some; more on this later) former *New York Times* book critic and essayist who died in 1990, fourteen months after he was diagnosed with prostate cancer. Two years later, his wife, Alexandra Broyard—as Lucy Kalanithi did for Paul more than twenty-five years later—compiled, edited, and published essays and journal notes by her husband, as well as a short story that chronicled Anatole's father's cancer and death, in the book *Intoxicated by My Illness*. The title thematizes Broyard's attempt to approach his illness at a slant, a wry sense of relationship with a disease that would ultimately kill him. And yet what irks him throughout these essays is less the cancer itself, horrid and painful as it is, than how the totalizing medicalization of illness contributes to a "diminished self." What diminishes him include the ways that cancer narrows the spectrum of relationality with others—"[My friends] are not intoxicated as I am by my illness, but sobered"—that turns him into a reluctant "existential hero."[18] So Broyard sets out in and through his writing to cultivate this sideways, alternative way of being sick, one that joins other emotions with the suffering that comes with living with cancer. Perhaps unsurprisingly but tellingly, he turns to the tools of criticism and writing to craft this differential self, one more expansive than the diminished medicalized one: "For it seems to me that every seriously ill person needs to develop a style for his illness. I think that only by insisting on your style can you keep from falling out of love with yourself as the illness attempts to diminish or disfigure you. . . . It may not be dying we fear so much, but the diminished self."[19] Illness as idiosyncratic style is less counterintuitive than at first glance, as illness under a medical gaze renders the person into the generic patient who must play, à la Parsons, the sick role whose only desire is to get better thanks to the work of the physician, who invariably becomes the protagonist even in the sick person's story. Broyard's ill style keeps him loveable, to himself and perhaps to the person with whom he is engaged in this intimate dance of health care, his doctor.

Turning to his physician, Broyard desires not the technical skill of medical service but a sensual pleasure from him (and the doctor is decidedly, always male; more on this later). Just as he imagines a more capacious landscape of desire in his ill world, so does Broyard want his physician to dwell in a desire that exceeds the scientific and, in the following case, gesture toward both the erotic and maternal: "I wouldn't demand a lot of my doctor's time: I just wish he would *brood* on my situation for perhaps five minutes, that he would give me his whole mind just once, be *bonded* with me for a brief space, survey my soul as well as my flesh, to get at my illness, for each man is ill in his own way."[20] To Broyard, intimacy from the physician provides a measure of singularity, which, in turn, enables pleasure that turns him into something more than a simple text of pathology: "I would also like a doctor who *enjoyed* me. I want to be a good story for him, to give him some of my art in exchange for his."[21] There is in this insistence on the aesthetic dimension of illness much of the book critic in Broyard; rendered a text, he grants his physician the role of critic yet doesn't yield critical agency completely. Even as he wishes his physician to "read" him with pleasure, Broyard must craft himself as a "good story," an interpretive and agentive enterprise that will provide the physician with an aesthetic experience that may supplement and even exceed the biomedical. He wishes his physician to engage in some version of reparative reading.

Broyard's memoiristic essays are emblematic of Frank's assertion that the bodies of the ill give shape to the narratives they tell of their illness: "People telling illness stories do not simply describe their sick bodies; their bodies give their stories their particular shape and direction."[22] Recognizing the ways that embodiment determines, even overdetermines, narrative is not particularly easy, given that we spend so much in human and other resources to reinforce narratives of able-bodiedness as the normative ones. "People certainly talk about their bodies in illness stories," Frank continues, "what is harder to hear in the story is the body creating the person."[23] The "good story" of Broyard's ill style, then, mandates his attention to the form of his essays, the transformation of his embodied experience through and into writing, from which he derives, as in his hope in his physician, some unexpected affirmative affects: "So much of a writer's life consists of assuming suffering, rhetorical suffering, that I felt something like relief, even elation, when the doctor told me that I had cancer of the prostate. Suddenly there was in the air a rich sense of crisis—real crisis, yet one that also contained echoes of ideas like the crisis of language, the crisis of literature, or of personality. It seemed to me that my existence, whatever I thought, felt, or did, had taken on a kind of meter, as in poetry or in taxis."[24] Form is connected to finitude: poetic meter will tell the time allotted in Broyard's life now marked by illness and the shadow of mortality. Illness establishes a relation between the body and the kind of narrative one needs to (re)tell in the story of this body. His prose must account for the urgency, but rather than a kind of panic, Broyard crafts a narrative of alacrity that forms his style. Dandied wit, as fanciful as Oscar Wilde, will make of his cancer a "good story" that doesn't require remission as its end, as it would not turn out to be after all. Instead, for Broyard, writing becomes the platform for his performance of the good story, for himself and for his audience, his physician: "Illness is primarily a drama, and it should be possible to enjoy it as well as to suffer it. I see now why the Romantics were so fond of illness—the sick man sees everything as metaphor. In this phase I'm infatuated with my cancer. It stinks of revelation."[25]

Yet for all the metaphors of desire and ironic attraction with which he suffuses his illness—infatuation, intoxication, fondness, revelation—ostensibly to be a good story for his doctor, Broyard's cultivation of his style in illness retains a curious monadism, almost solipsistic in its insistence on his singularity that seems to preclude the very sociality he claims to want in his relationship with his physician. Throughout his essays, Broyard rarely regards the condition of other ill people, fellow sufferers in the hospital, except to note his class (but, significantly, not racial) difference from them. There is something affectively guarded in his captivation by *his* desire that prevents him from imagining the desire of others, whether other patients or even his physician; he fantasizes, remember, his doctor's desire as one of "brooding" over him. And one can't help but insert into this particular stylization of illness—so whimsical, on the one hand ("stinks of revelation"), and so authoritarian, on the other ("illness is primarily a drama")—the guardedness with which Broyard kept other dimensions of his identity at bay, the open secret of his Black family that he disavowed throughout his life and career. These essays are simultaneously "stinking" revelations of illness and of unrevealed racial passing. In his trenchant profile of Broyard for the *New Yorker*, sardonically titled "White like Me," Henry Louis Gates Jr. notes a similar reserve in the manner that Broyard conducted himself as he vaulted to the heights of the literary world, his racial shadow always lurking but never visible: "There could be no relaxation of vigilance: in his most intimate relationships, there were guardrails."[26] To this Gates offers a rather brutal diagnostic of Broyard's disavowal: "Broyard passed not because he thought that race wasn't important but because he knew that it was. The durable social facts of race were beyond reason, and . . . their strength came at the expense of style. . . . For his part, he wasn't taking any chances. At a certain point, he seems to have decided that all he had to do was stay white and die."[27]

In one of the essays on illness, titled "Toward a Literature on Illness," Broyard perhaps unwittingly, maybe subtly, invokes a penchant for the racially particular in his assertion for an illness style, "other strategies beside medical ones," when he describes the following scene as an ideal expression of this desired style: "I saw on television an Afro-Cuban band playing in the streets of Spanish Harlem. It was a very good band, and before long a man stepped out of the crowd and began dancing. He was very good, too, even though he had only one leg and was dancing on crutches. He danced on those crutches as other people dance on ice skates, and I think that there's probably a 'dance' for every condition. As Kenneth Burke, one of our best literary critics, said, the symbolic act is the dancing of an attitude."[28] Broyard's momentary identification with, presumably, a disabled man of color and his dance as a mode of living his condition through the performance of dance takes on Burkean symbolic action, something that comes awfully close to perlocutionary force to this most raced of instances in his essay. And yet immediately afterward, Broyard writes: "As a preparation for writing, as a first step toward evolving a strategy for my illness, I've begun to take tap-dancing lessons, something I've always wanted to do."[29] Metaphor materializes into actual dancing, and Broyard's choice of dance genre is telling. As Constance Valis Hill argues in *Tap Dancing America*, tap dancing derives its origins from both Black and African vernacular performance and Irish immigrant jigs. Yet its popular Hollywood heyday, ensconced in the white mythologies of the Fred Astaire and Gene Kelly decades of the 1940s and 1950s, obscures the ways that tap's innovative, improvisational performance came from longstanding development of the form by African American dancers, with jazz tap dance as the "form of expressive production that led to a specifically African American modernism."[30] The turn from Afro-Cuban sounds and the image of a disabled man of color to an unspecified pedagogy of tap dancing constitutes a significant flattening of desire and suggests the extent to which his "good story" is narrower than he might intend.

Sister Outsider: Audre Lorde's *Cancer Journals*

Broyard's careful style that derives from his anxieties around racial reckoning, which, in turn, circumscribes what he allows himself to enjoy, limits his ability to see in his guild the fellow travelers of illness. He maintains that "[sick people] also need a literature of their own. Misery loves company—if it's good company," but then remarks, "Surprisingly enough, there isn't much good company in this rapidly proliferating field. A critical illness is one of our momentous experiences, yet I haven't seen a single nonfiction book that does it justice."[31] Broyard then provides a litany of writers, some physicians, some novelists, *most of them men* (with the exception of Natalie Spingarm, a journalist whom he castigates for being too clinical, and Susan Sontag's well-known polemic *Illness as Metaphor*), with whom he disagrees. Striking here is the complete omission of the fledging but significant archive of cancer memoirs written primarily by women. Betty Rollin's was among the first; of them, Audre Lorde's *The Cancer Journals* is probably the most durably famous, in print since its first publication in 1980.

"This is work I must do alone," writes Lorde, which mirrors the loneliness of Broyard's "existential hero." Yet whereas Broyard sublimates the solitude forced on him by his ill body by developing a fanciful style that gives him the space to "play" with his cancer (and his doctor), in part also to distract from the equally hard kernels of his closeted racial identity, Lorde approaches her "ill style" as one of utter exposure and visibility, an embrace of social identity likely anathema to Broyard. "Off and on," she writes, "I kept thinking. I have cancer. I'm a black lesbian feminist poet, how am I going to do this now? Where are the models for what I'm supposed to be in this situation? But there were none. This is it, Audre. You're on your own."[32] Like our contemporary Asian Americans' dilemma, Lorde cannot find a model with whom to write about what she thinks about "off and on," and like Broyard, she seeks the "good company" of other sick people. But for Lorde, "good company" would involve women like her: Black, feminist, lesbian writers, all expressions of identity that Broyard would rather expunge or regard as too particular. Lorde's desire to search for models is an insistence that her identity is as universal as one that disavows a racial identity other than white.

Broyard searches for a literature of illness to tend to his existential loneliness, but Lorde looks to her immediate network of lovers and friends, her "sisterhood" that tends to her bodily and emotional needs as they come, a realized feminist practice of care that she juxtaposes with the cruelty of medical staff. She recalls:

> Our friends came and were there, loving and helpful and there, brought coats to pile upon my bed and then a comforter and blankets because the hospital had no spare blankets, they said, and I was so desperately chilled from the cold recovery room. I remember their faces as we shared the knowledge and the promise of shared strength in the trial days to come. In some way it was as if each of the people

I love most dearly came one by one to my bedside where we made a silent pledge of strength and sisterhood no less sacred than if it had been pledged in blood rather than love.[33]

After her mastectomy, Lorde provides a litany of these friends, naming them as if to both individuate them and weave them into a network of intersubjective mutuality: "From the time I woke up to the slow growing warmth of Adrienne's and Bernice's and Deanna's and Michelle's and Frances' coats on the bed, I felt Beth Israel Hospital wrapped in a web of woman love and strong wishes of faith and hope for the whole time I was there, and it made self-healing more possible, knowing I was not alone. Throughout the hospitalization and for some time after, it seemed that no problem was too small or too large to be shared and handled."[34] The warmth literally and figuratively provided by the company and coats of her friends contrasts sharply with the coldness of the hospital and those paid and charged to care for Lorde professionally. Rarely are medical staff kind to her, an understated insinuation of racism, sexism, and homophobia that disregards Lorde's somatic condition and her desire to voice its suffering: "I remember screaming and cursing with pain in the recovery room, and I remember a disgusted nurse giving me a shot. I remember a voice telling me to be quiet because there were sick people here, and my saying, well, I have a right, because I'm sick too."[35] This contrast, from the care of her friends to the revulsion of the nurse, that results in the silencing of Lorde from articulating her pain registers both the divides that she experiences between the medical "care" of her mastectomy and the healing of the coats and presence, as well as the difficulty of giving voice to the condition that she suffers. Lorde identifies her illness as constitutive of her identity, just as much as the other elements that make up who she is, a coming to terms with the new contours of her body. In doing this, she also allows her body to register the unconscious racist bias that health-care staff reveal in their refusal to recognize in this Black woman pain and suffering, a bias that remains durably endemic to this day.[36]

Elizabeth Alexander sums up the challenge that Lorde thus undertakes in this telling: "In Lorde's work, the body speaks its own history; she chooses corporeal language to articulate what she could not previously put into words."[37] What always threatens is the silence expected of women with breast cancer—most notably, in the insistence that they, Lorde included, wear a prosthesis to cover up the effects of mastectomy. The prosthetic breast allows a woman to "pass" as someone who does not bear the wounds of cancer and maintains the fiction of able-bodiedness and health. Lorde wants none of this: "It is that very difference [of cancer] that I wish to affirm, because I have lived it, and survived it, and wish to share that strength with other women."[38] It is indeed silence, like the invisibility that is the imperative of prosthesis, that Lorde ultimately demands to break, for it is silence that prevents women from discerning what new voice and story emerge from their bodies altered by cancer. "May these words serve as encouragement for other women to speak and to act out of our experiences with cancer and with other threats of death," she writes, "for silence has never brought us anything of worth. Most of all, may these words underline the possibilities of self-healing and the richness of living for all women."[39]

So Lorde's memoir sets out to create a different style, even a form, of life writing that Cynthia Wu describes as eschewing discrete binarisms of public and private, formal and informal, rational and affective. "Lorde harnesses the potential of revealing the 'private,' and 'personal,'" writes Wu:

> The unveiling of the incidents surrounding her illness turns the private material of daily life into a political tool that encourages public discussion among women who are dealing with cancer, a topic that has traditionally been shrouded in silence and secrecy. Her text is a collection of diary entries interspersed with writings in other genres such as the essay and the poem, and this arrangement of her writings is strategic. Topically relevant journal entries appear immediately before or after polemical essays, and the union of the two genres creates a doublepronged argument that yokes the private and the public sphere.[40]

Late in the memoir, Lorde records a journal entry during which she wonders how her illness has transformed her sense of temporality, from "counting the milliseconds" of her days to contemplating her inevitable end, whether because of cancer or otherwise: "For once we accept the actual existence of our dying, who can ever have power over us again?"[41] She then moves (back) into essay mode, her journal query now rich fodder not only for her own reflection but for the intimate public she cultivates through her writing as a wounded storyteller: "I am writing this now in a new year, recalling, trying to piece together that chunk of my recent past, so that I, or anyone else in need or desire, can dip into it at will if necessary to find the ingredients with which to build a wider construct. That is an important function of the telling of experience."[42] Nothing about her experience or in the telling of it is ideal. She was ill and remains wounded and will have died some twelve years after the release of *The Cancer Journals*. The perfectibility that Kalanithi so sought before his own illness is a world away for Lorde. But, as Frank notes, "Lorde not only can live with that imperfection, but she also offers it as a basis of affiliation with others."[43]

Broyard's and Lorde's memoirs ceaselessly strive not for perfection or even for restitution (though both allude to hope for remission). Instead, they strive toward a writing practice of telling the story of their ill bodies as good stories. Of course, the two differ in what counts as good. Broyard searches for language that plays with the revelatory stink of his cancer, words that keep him alive and present to himself when pain and medicalization threaten to overwhelm. Lorde reaches out beyond the scope of the medical staff and toward the (Black, lesbian, feminist) women she loves and into herself to reanimate her erotic self, to love her altered body anew, and to call on women to communicate with one another about their wounds. I have chosen these two non–Asian American illness stories as a prelude to the Asian American ones because of the range of their ill style, from the angled and charged, yet ultimately closeted, prose of Broyard to the stridently vocal and visible rhetorical politics of Lorde. Both present a deliberate crafting of style constitutive of their raced, gendered ill bodies, a condition with which, frankly, all writers must contend (including white and male writers, their objections notwithstanding). It's a narrative dilemma that Asian Americans, given that their tradition of illness literature must emerge practically ex nihilo, must especially develop with heightened intention. What Broyard and Lorde point to as we approach Asian American storytellers is that each of them must become a style crafter and model writer; each is her or his own existential hero; each has to do the work alone. Call this, perhaps, the iconoclasm of illness.

Cancer and Leftist Ableism: Fred Ho

Fred Ho's style is evident in the prologue of *Diary of a Radical Cancer Warrior*, in which he concludes a self-referential apologia with the figuration of himself as a warrior instead of a mere survivor/victim of cancer.* It contains a characteristically long-winded sentence that illuminates the stakes that Ho lays out for a narrative that chronicles his experiences and struggles with colorectal cancer and its treatment, stakes distilled in the subtitle of the book, "Fighting Cancer and Capitalism at the Cellular Level." The lines read: "Make no mistake: this is a war to the end, an end to which success or failure depends on how much we make ourselves to be the principled warriors

---

* I need to say here that stories of Ho's sexually assaulting, harassing, and stalking women exist and that I believe them. This does not change my reading of his memoir; but rather, it informs it.

in seeking solutions and not compromises to our personal health, wellness, transformation, and to curing the planet once and for all of the greatest threat to life itself."[44] Ho will return again and again to this extended metaphor of warfare, and of himself as a cancer warrior, throughout his memoir, even as the modalities of war making against his disease shift dramatically about two-thirds of the way into the book. After his cancer returns for the fourth time, Ho rejects all medical treatment and turns exclusively to naturopathic modes of therapy. By the book's end, he claims, he has "completely reject[ed] the notion of a complementary medicine."[45] Thus, Ho's stance as a principled warrior figures his enemy—by the end of the book and, presumably, his life (he died in 2014)—to be not only the cancer that afflicts him but also the biomedical regime that he'd earlier marshaled for his war against cancer, but that he now views not only as no longer a solution but as yet another problem in the deep imbrication of cancer and capitalism.

Ho's narrative filtering of his experience of cancer and medical treatment as a form of warfare is both mundane and significant. It's mundane in part because this discourse around cancer and warfare has had a fairly long, if recent, history. While he mentions it nowhere in his book, the idea that cancer should be fought as one would fight a war has its origins in the United States during the mid- to late 1960s, when medical practitioners began to develop new protocols of chemotherapy to treat what were until then fatal and heartbreaking diagnoses of childhood leukemia.[46] In the wake of some therapeutic successes, leading cancer researchers and wealthy elites hoped to mobilize the resources and scale of the federal government to move expeditiously in finding a "cure" for cancer. On December 9, 1969, a group called the Citizens Committee for the Conquest of Cancer took out a full-page ad in the *New York Times* that read: "Mr. Nixon, you can cure cancer."[47] A bill passed overwhelmingly in Congress, and on December 23, 1971, President Richard Nixon signed the National Cancer Act, which allocated $1.5 billion over three years (almost $10 billion in 2017 dollars), an act that journalists quickly dubbed the "president's personal war on cancer."[48] The use of warfare rhetoric to enact social policy is a hallmark of twentieth-century marshaling of national resources that speaks to the ways that actual warfare was one of the few ways that national policy and, more important, transformations in state structures and resources took place. Warfare turns policy into patriotic practice. But as Susan Sontag points out in her classic essay "Illness as Metaphor" (1978), while warfare has been a controlling metaphor in descriptions of cancer and its treatments, its variety of distortions by way of military language gives its depiction a speculative dimension: "Cancer is being magnified and projected into a metaphor for the biggest enemy, the furthest goal. Thus,

Nixon's bid to match Kennedy's promise to put Americans on the moon was, appropriately enough, the promise to 'conquer' cancer. Both were science-fiction ventures."[49] Its scope and scale perhaps help us also to understand how much such language suffuses micro-level, individuated relations and experiences that turn phrases such as "died after a long battle with cancer" or "we will fight this cancer together" into common parlance.

Ho's usage is significant from the sheer fact that, as mundane as the metaphor is, his book remains the first published account of cancer written by an Asian American, a milestone made possible by his notoriety within leftist circles.[50] His biography is well known in Asian American studies, but let me briefly rehearse: born in Amherst, Massachusetts, and the son of a college professor, Ho sought out in his adolescence alternative political identities to counter his personal experiences of white racism. When the Nation of Islam briefly opened membership to non-Black people, Ho was among the first to join. Later, he joined the Asian American revolutionary group I Wor Kuen (IWK), which embraced Marxism-Leninism and modeled itself after the Black Panther Party.[51] Over the next four decades, Ho sought to mobilize his training as a jazz musician to develop an Asian American artistic sensibility and cofounded the Afro Asian Music Ensemble, a platform that could serve as a cultural component to revolutionary activity and that paralleled, borrowed from, and appropriated elements of the larger and longer Black jazz and arts tradition. Coterminous with his forays into music and performance is an eclectic portfolio of writings that range from meditations on the political possibilities of jazz to Asian American radical politics and identity.[52] What has remained durably consistent throughout his career is an unapologetic didacticism and an investment in cultural vanguardism that his admirers cherish and his detractors find simplistic, even vulgar and elitist.

Ho began writing about his experience with cancer on several online sites shortly after his diagnosis, including on his Myspace page, but in 2011 he agreed to curate his cancer diaries into book form in the hope that he might reach a wider audience. In his penultimate entry, Ho explicitly addresses his reasons for writing and disseminating the diary for public consumption—as he puts it, "present [it] in real time, to show the journey and development, the twists and turns, the mistakes, the failings, the transformations, and the lessons."[53] In book form, the text meanders through the vicissitudes of an aggressive and ultimately fatal disease, during which Ho documents in detail the consequences of surgery and chemotherapy, including considerable bouts of diarrhea, fatigue, and sexual impotence. At other moments, Ho transcribes medical narratives of him as the patient and splices in short essays and eulogies of friends and letters written to him by fans, admirers, and mentees. As a narrative, it doesn't follow an epiphanic quest story that typifies many cancer memoirs but, instead, moves between the quotidian gross and the philosophically utopian, though there is a phantasm of miraculous cure that haunts the book throughout.

If there is a conceptual anchor to the diary, it is Ho's attempt to map a political reading onto the horrors of his experience as a cancer warrior, one who first fights cancer and later fights both the disease and allopathic medicine. Throughout the book, passages such as this early one frame the more mundane descriptions of daily life: "I am daily convinced that fighting cancer is a war. It is a war fought on the medical/cellular level, it is a war fought on the social-economic-political level against the U.S. HMO system of profiteering off healthcare, and it is a war fought on the spiritual-physical-mental-manual level of yin-yang."[54] Later Ho returns to the deep connection between his fight against cancer as a personal mode of resistance against the malignant forces of capitalism: "The war will continue for a long time, not only for me personally to make sure no cancer cells ever grow again inside of me, but to support the ongoing greater war to remove the cancer of capitalism from this world."[55] Such passages typify Ho's recursive strategy to wrest political meaning out of his suffering, which augment each time the cancer returns until, after cancer returns the fourth time following a brief year of remission, Ho turns on the biomedical regime on which he had relied, albeit with some measure of ambivalence for its profit motive. "Mainstream medicine is the succubus," Ho opines late in the book. "While you are in repose, believing it to be there for your best interests, it is in reality functioning according to its own logic, which inevitably is to facilitate the interests of capitalism (profits), all the while convincing you, along with its practitioners (many of whom are well intentioned), that it is healing you when indeed it is not and, often, making you sicker."[56] Thus, his personal struggle with cancer and, later, his decision to reject allopathic medical technologies constitute nothing less than his contribution to this war, a form of activism that demonstrates that autonomy from what he calls the "teratogenic-carcinogenic-iatrogenic matrix" will facilitate well-being and healing, which includes, tentatively, a hoped-for but never realized cure.

But this hoped-for yet never realized cure, like his insistence on cultivating his warrior's style—both a commitment to healing *as* an operation against the degradations of cancer, medicine, and capitalism—relies on ableist assumptions of activism that presume health, wholeness, and the restored body as the marker of transcendence over the evils of capitalism and cancer. Throughout the book Ho insists that a new treatment or regime will be the one to help him "beat cancer," one that he increasingly pins on his desire to assume complete control of his health care. When he breaks with allopathic treatment,

Ho insists, again recursively, on what he calls a "no compromise manifesto" which includes the top priority of leading his own treatment; later, in a letter to his sister who also experienced cancer twice, Ho recounts, "I am for the first time in the cancer war, truly free and feel great because I'm in charge."[57] In this assertion of freedom Ho notes his restoration to health: the lowering of his blood pressure, the alleviation of his neuropathy, the partial return of his sexual function, and his considerable loss of weight.[58] His assertion of freedom as individuation, made manifest by his daily individual actions of naturopathic self-improvement, depend largely on an attachment to what Tobin Siebers calls an ideology of ability, which at its core is a barely acknowledged faith in the restorability and perfectibility of the body.[59] To this extent, warrior activism rests on a fundamental belief in bodily and narrative restitution, an ethos with which Ho closes his narrative when he is asked how to receive a cancer diagnosis. "You can think of it as a horrific curse," Ho concludes, or "you can take it as a gift, an opportunity to change yourself *forever*, to never go back to the carcinogenic matrix of the life you once lived, and to build a new person and new life that is truly better!"[60] Ho's exclamatory tone, as if yelling at himself, as well as at you, enlists a rhetoric of cure that is built into those that populate cancer center brochures and hospital billboards. My institution, for example, dubs itself simply "Anti-Cancer"; a recent television advertisement for the Dana-Farber Cancer Institute has it "Cracking the Code" (presumably, of cancer genes).[61]

This notion of cancer as a gift is not unique to cancer memoirs, but given Ho's particular iteration of cancer as a bodily signifier of global capitalism and the way forward to treat and fight one's cancer—to assert control over one's treatment, to cultivate the body by optimizing its intakes—creates a strange and ironic correlation between Ho's leftist ableism and contemporary neoliberal notions of the care of the self.[62] Ho's final call to change yourself "forever," this never-ending cultivation of the self precisely at the moment one is no longer reliant on something that might approximate institutional or civic life, imagines warrior life as a life that demands a commitment to the utopian as perfectible and to an autonomy that, to return to the significance of this text as a first by an Asian American, welcomes back the specter of the model minority that continues to haunt contemporary Asian American stories.

What is strangely but perhaps not surprisingly missing from this extended meditation on a struggle with cancer as warfare is a well-trodden genealogy offered by Lorde in *The Cancer Journals*, written less than a decade after Nixon's War on Cancer. Lorde insisted that the silence she encountered within breast cancer circles was a systemically shared suffering and vulnerability, one that demanded a rhetorical and identitarian transformation from cancer victim to cancer warrior. In inveighing against the assumption that women who had received mastectomies should wear breast prosthetics so as not to make others uncomfortable, Lorde reminds her readers that Moshe Dayan, then the prime minister of Israel, wore an eyepatch for a lost eye. She recounts: "The world sees him as a warrior with an honorable wound, and a loss of a piece of himself which he has marked, and mourned, and moved beyond."[63] Lorde extends this metaphor of the wounded, vulnerable warrior to herself and other women: "Well, women with breast cancer are warriors, also. I have been to war, and still am. . . . For me, my scars are an honorable reminder that I may be a casualty in the cosmic war against radiation, animal fat, air pollution, Mc-Donald's hamburgers and Red Dye No. 2, but the fight is still going on, and I am still a part of it."[64] Lorde calls attention to her wounded body not as one that is perfectible, but as a vulnerable, contingent body that is still meaning-ful, and meaningful precisely in its shared vulnerability with others similarly afflicted. Why Ho seems not to have read Lorde's vision of warrior identity remains open and curious, given his repeated public commitments to what he calls "matriarchal socialism" as a corrective to patriarchal capitalism.[65] (This is not to mention what is at stake in this shared investment in imagining cancer as warfare as opposed to, say, coexistence.[66]) But something tells me that the possessive attachments to control, autonomy, and ableism that undergird his activism prevent Ho from imagining the possibility that simply bearing wit-ness to his fellow cancer survivors—including those who die—might offer a far more radical and, dare I say, utopian vision of sociality that might decide that simply being a community of wounded storytellers is just fine.[67]

Illness and Intersubjectivity: Brandy Liên Worrall

While not anywhere near a place resembling utopia, Brandy Liên Worrall's memoir chronicles an assemblage born of her bodily woundedness. At first glance, there seems little room for Worrall to listen to what her body tells, buffeted as she is by sets of expectations that are legion. Her narrative hurtles through time and space as she reveals her travails as the rebellious daugh-ter of a Vietnamese immigrant mother and Vietnam War veteran father; as a long-suffering wife of an Asian American studies professor, from whom she'll be divorced; as a devoted but harrowed mother of two children and, later, a third child; and, perhaps most important for our purposes, a formerly healthy person turned ill person and, throughout much of the book, a patient suffering from breast cancer and its attendant therapies. There are certainly vestiges of fantasies of familial bliss peppered throughout the memoir: of her youthful crush on a young, charismatic professor that results in marriage and children; of her jet-setting brother-in-law delivering lectures on cutting-edge architecture while playing in amateur hockey leagues. But Worrall's narrative opens abruptly: "Things are not fun right now. In fact, they kinda suck."[68] And with that, we are invited to journey with her into her maelstrom of familial and somatic chaos. By the end of the first chapter, we already have foreshadowing of a marriage in shambles, her brother-in-law dead from lung cancer. In the immediate moments after her cancer diagnosis, Worrall offers a glimpse of what Ronald Dworkin calls a "narrative wreck," an unmooring of narrative stability in which sensory processes are both overloaded and unable to register.[69] Standing with Charles, her husband, on a corner in Vancouver and finding it impossible to figure out where to go—literally and figuratively—Worrall recounts: "The atmosphere suddenly became so foreign, everything with its vitality, unaware of or unconcerned with my diagnosis."[70] Here, Worrall's sense of complete discombobulation echoes Frank's observation that illness disrupts a fundamental component of how people tell their stories, which is a capacity for temporality. "The conventional expectation of any narrative," Frank writes, "held alike by listeners and storytellers, is for a past that leads into a present that sets in place a foreseeable future."[71] By contrast, Frank continues, "the illness story is [narratively] wrecked because its present is not what the past was supposed to lead up to, and the future is scarcely thinkable."[72] For Worrall, the scarcely thinkable future is exacerbated by the divergent temporalities that she and Charles live, increasingly so when she begins her chemotherapy. "My life," she writes, "has come to sudden halt. . . . But Charles just keeps on going. My cancer is shitty timing for him. He's got this huge blockbuster conference in a couple of weeks, so he's at meetings and press conferences nonstop. . . . No, life hasn't come to a halt. Rather, it's being lived out in spite of me."[73] Of course, it is neither that Worrall's life has halted nor that life is being lived out in spite of her, but instead that her life, now suffused with illness, operates on a differential temporality and geography from her still abled-bodied, healthy husband's. Ill time is "shitty" for Charles; ill time is time lived out of spite for the healthy body. Likewise, while Charles shuttles across Vancouver, from home to school, and moves transnationally and globally as he builds his professional reputation, Worrall's circuit is demonstrably more constrained between home and clinic. Indeed, it is the divergent physical journeys between the two—the clinic becoming more Worrall's home than their shared house, Charles reluctantly traveling with her for chemotherapy when he is not tethered to his work obligations—that further highlight how "unhomely" the home life has become. Worrall's vulnerable condition makes intolerable the capacity for Charles to live his ambitious futurity. Later, Charles will have an affair that will break up the marriage for good, but throughout the narrative, the signs that the two are in different geographies and temporalities, and speak increasingly different languages, deepening their mutual alienation, become visible well before the actual infidelity takes place.

But to the extent that her cancer wrecks whatever fantasy of a life she may have held with Charles, Worrall's illness also opens her to wholly unexpected and unimagined ways to connect, particularly with her parents. Temporalities and geographies of vulnerability open channels of communicability heretofore unknown to Worrall. While the squabbling persists throughout the memoir, particularly between daughter and mother, the narrative also makes clear that new capacities for relation emerge, a kind of shared suffering. For example, in the passage in which she describes the atmosphere as foreign, figuratively a different country, shortly after her diagnosis, Worrall immediately recalls her mother's illness upon her arrival to the United States, both the result of experiencing a Pennsylvania winter for the first time and the loss and isolation born of displacement from Vietnam. "[My mother] told me of how she struggled," Worrall reflects, "how she almost died the first few months there, how she wanted badly to go home. She crossed the divide, and it was the hardest thing she'd ever done. That's when her new normal began. I understand now, Mom, the divide. The harsh precipice between there and here, then and now."[74] Later, as she awaits reconstructive surgery following a mastectomy, Worrall recounts her father's struggles with drug and alcohol addiction, his going in and out of rehab programs at the local Veterans Administration hospital, and his lingering post-traumatic stress disorder to which she now relates as someone "who's been through the shit."[75] Worrall even reconnects to her former child self as a young girl who suffered epileptic mal seizures. Her ill and wounded body, the somatic site of her distance from Charles, also becomes the mode through which she enlivens the stories of her parents, whom she regards at the beginning of the memoir as, respectively, a "Crazy Asian Mother" and a "handful" of a father. Her narrative of illness slides into their stories, so that chapters structurally become recursive narrative occasions: a moment at a doctor's office, a procedure, or a particularly bad evening triggers an episode of her mother's struggles in Vietnam or her father's recounting of war horror. Her parents' stories help fill in hers.

Indeed, early in her memoir she recounts a recurring sequence of dreams, what she calls her "Vietnam War dreams," even as she also notes that her parents seldom talked about their experiences of the war. Yet in her "chemo haze," Worrall can no longer discern whether she has awoken from a dream hued by an "orange-red aura" with the smell of "singed skin": "The chemical smell and taste biting the insides of my nose, mouth, and throat make me wonder if Mom and Dad had the same assault on their senses when they breathed in the Agent Orange that was so casually dropped from planes flying overhead."[76] Of course, the extent to which the U.S. military has been, and continues to be, dismissive of those exposed to the slow violence of its chemical warfare program is well documented.[77] But here Worrall suggests not only that she receives a traumatic postmemory, but that she is the recipient of an intergenerational poison. "See those bright trees suddenly dropping dead?" Worrall muses sardonically. "Nothing to worry about. Later: see those babies being born without limbs? Nothing to worry about. See those vets dying of prostate cancer in alarming numbers? Nothing to worry about. Stuff happens. See me getting poisoned so I can get rid of this inexplicable cancer? Nothing to worry about."[78] Agent Orange is passed from parent to child and, perhaps most ironically, as both disease and cure, insofar as the cancer is an expression of the herbicide and as the chemotherapy constitutes an animacy related to Agent Orange: chemical agents that may have caused her cancer are now being called on to cure her of her illness. Worrall thus sees in her parents a shared toxicity. Even as cancer is an unqualified horror that speaks to shared trauma, illness becomes a mode through which a differential Asian Americanness might emerge, one determined by legacies of warfare and militarized poison that are somatically lived rather than intellectually imagined. In this way, the more legibly political identity—Charles, the studious Asian American studies professor—is less aware of its complicity in the institutions that damaged Worrall and her parents.

Worrall enacts what is possible when illness is neither avoided nor romanticized but fully engaged, the experience put to use toward relational means and ends. This gesture of reaching toward others, desire born of distinctive but mutual bodily contingencies, makes the memoir not only the story of Worrall's struggle with cancer but also an intersubjective familial narrative that frames the Asian American and her family far from the capitalist enterprise of model minority fantasy. Indeed, Worrall's narrative suggests that this familial fantasy—one that was barely available to her, in which she was expected to live out the life of the daughter bound by debt to her multiracial parents—not only would not have been helpful in her illness but might very well have destroyed her utterly had she been wedded to it. Instead, it is out of the wounds of her deeply flawed, troubled, and broken family that new modes of sociality are made possible, which should remind us of what Mel Chen has written about regarding an animated relationship to toxicity that "propels queer loves, especially once we release it from exclusively human hosts, disproportionately inviting dis/ability, industrial labor, biological targets, and military vaccine recipients—inviting loss and its 'losers' and trespassing containers of animacy."[79] Perhaps less utopian than Chen's vision,

Worrall's reimagined relationality is still an opening that guarantees nothing but binds her across space and time, reaching toward a desire shared even by those who are now dead.[80]

Digital Recursions: Blogging Illness

A brief excursus from illness memoirs to reach back into their proto-form. I mentioned that Ho began writing about his cancer on a Myspace page. Much of Worrall's memoir has an earlier version from a blog that she started on July 16, 2007, and on which she still occasionally posts (though considerably less since 2009; it was in 2007 and 2008 that she wrote most prolifically on the blog). Titled "Cancer Fucking Sucks," Worrall's blog site chronicles, from the moment of her diagnosis, the difficult and lonely, alienating journey into the ontologically different world of illness, even as she struggles to maintain the quotidian daily activities of motherhood and conjugal partnership and moments of levity and even pleasure. Her first post, "Diagnosis: Damn," in which she announces the diagnosis of breast cancer, records her feeling toward cancer as a terribly inconvenient interruption to life: "I'm 31 years old. I've got two kids, and I've got a ton of shit to do. Last thing I need is cancer. It's the last thing anyone needs. . . . None of this makes any sense. So yeah, like the URL says, cancer fucking sucks."[81] As if to demonstrate the non-sense of confronting illness, the blog entry received no comments; even in 2019, some twelve years after she posted her diagnosis for the world to witness (and the last time I checked), not one person had mustered the ability to respond to Worrall's descent. Over time, however, subsequent posts would find readers, interlocutors who often try to drop words of encouragement or of empathy/sympathy regarding particularly difficult travails. Over time, Worrall would write in anticipation of regular readers, as in her August 19, 2008, entry, "Not-so-Dead Arm," which begins, "First, I want to thank everyone for keeping up with my blog, even when I haven't been so good at keeping up with it myself. You know how yappy I've been. . . . [W]ell it seems that the recovery process has been silencing me."[82] The rest of this entry, about the multistage process of breast reconstruction and other dimensions of her recovery, prompts some of her regular readers to respond jokingly about the size and beauty of her reconstructed breasts ("wow . . . brand new boobies . . . i'm excited to meet the new girls :-)").

The new media and digital media critic Geert Lovink regards the blog rather critically as a form or genre that produces what he calls a "distributed subjectivity," by which he seeks to underscore, on the one hand, the radical individuality of self-expression that bloggers perform even as, on the other, they are situated in a network of other bloggers, readers, and users of digital platforms, "part of an existing social network . . . simply nodes created to store material."[83] Blogs, for Lovink, are instances of the doleful features of contemporary digital life, distributed subjectivities that are little more than capitalist hall passes for expressive egoism: "The personal that is produced for display uncouples from any supposition of a true or underlying self. . . . What matters is what appears. Communicative capitalism is not an identity container. Rather, people produce their identities through networked communications media. The internet is the medium for mass experience, but one that is highly differentiated and singularized. Blogging comes in as the technology of that experience."[84]

As expressions of the ordinary reaching for and aspiring to the celebrity, blogs allegorize the ways that new media reproduces the alienating effects of capitalist endeavors for extraction and abstraction, according to Lovink. He's not wrong, but he's also not complete in his assessment. Within the embedded algorithms of Google (which owns the Blogger platform that Worrall uses), much of which continue to gather data from her and her readers to facilitate value-added forms of advertisement and monetization (for the company, not for Worrall or you and me), there is in each entry, no better expressed than in her first, a cry that hurtles into the digital abyss and wonders whether someone might hear it on the other side of the technological looking glass. Even data sets are tied to wounded bodies, and, as Fred Moten might remind us, (humans as) things have social lives that may be beyond capitalist recognition.[85] Digital platforms may hold captive distributed subjectivities of bloggers *and* be the form or genre through which something differentially networked might emerge to communicate to someone like Worrall at her end of a WiFi signal that her words have reached another's hippocampus.

Can we deign to call this distributed subjectivity also, at least sometimes, a community? Jennifer Ho thinks so. In her reading of the role that the blog has played in the contemporary cultivation of Asian adoptee identity, she insists that blogs are generically a communal form: "Blogs do not exist in a vacuum: they are connected to other blogs, and they form a network and a community. . . . Community is also what lies at the heart of the identities of adult adoptee bloggers, and community is the means by which they create their own stories that challenge the traditional sentimental narratives of adoption through an embrace of racial ambiguity."[86] The community of Asian adoptees in the United States and beyond that has emerged in the past quarter-century is directly correlated to the abilities of these people to discover and discern shared stories out of their relative and respective isolation via digital interactions of blogging and other forms of social media.[87] "The importance of shared community that the blogs represent," Ho continues, "cannot be overstated." This, of course runs the risk of over-romanticizing these forma-tions, if one were to ignore Lovink's caveats.[88] We will heed both—Lovink's caveat of the internet as blog turning us into thingly commodities and Ho's celebration of blogs as a way for profoundly isolated and lonely people to find other equally lonely and isolated people, to feel less miserable and, perhaps, find something joyfully requited.

Jennifer Ho herself would turn to the blog form when in April 2010, she, too, was diagnosed with breast cancer. Her blog, *No F****** Pink Ribbons*, was active for three years, during which she narrated the vicissitudes and messiness of ill life: one that she survived, but also one from which she would never return to a former, able-bodied self. At several points during her treat-ment, Ho feels like a thing—all patients with life-threatening illness do—so the impulse to narrate this feeling of thingliness, of the struggle to discern a self as she is subjected to thingly patienthood, serves to open her to desire to listen to other stories of those who have lived with breast cancer. In her penultimate entry, she recounts with a certain amount of surprise, "I didn't realize how much I wanted to be with other women who had experienced breast cancer."[89] Fiber optic and wireless connections provide companies such as Google vital data about Ho and her readers; it also provides the ability for Ho to be in conversation with other cancer blog authors and advocates, as one would see in her August 7, 2012, entry, when she is contacted by a blog devoted to those with mesothelioma.[90] It is a network—perhaps even a rhizome—of suffering, but one that conditions its writers and readers that something like illness, a form of living, is teleological only if one still believes the fantasy of restorable health. For everyone else, there is the circumscribed condition of distributed (inter)subjectivities that helps make their vulnerable lives a bit more bearable. Or, as Ho writes about the adoptee blog form (and very well could about her own ill blog genre), "[This] is one of the reasons that the blogs written by [Asian Americans living with cancer] become a powerful medium for charting the negotiation of this ambiguity. Blogs do not have closure or resolution; they are ongoing testimonials of their writers. They are interactive forms of communication that create a living community of other [people living with and dying from illness]. For [Asian Americans living with cancer,] there cannot be closure because the mourning and loss that they feel over their [illness] is continuous."[91]

Unlike Worrall or Jennifer Ho, who created their blogs to write out and through their experience with cancer and subsequent treatment, Christine

Hyung-Oak Lee began hers not as an illness blog but as a medium through which she could journal while composing a novel and completing a master of fine arts at Mills College. In September 2006, Lee transitioned into the pseudonymous blog jadepark.wordpress.com in large part to avoid an online male harasser who had been trolling her eponymous blog. Throughout the fall, her posts consisted of a range of topics, from books she was currently reading and her frustration with being overshadowed by her husband to a quirky obsession with Doritos. Early on, there's an admission of compulsion toward busyness that, Lee wonders, might need future attention: "Being industrious is a value pounded into me. 'Get off the couch!' was a popular refrain in my childhood household. To spend every minute of a day being productive was lauded. To minimize sleep was an honor. But what of relaxing? I ought to do some more of that. I've come to realize that relaxing is a much more challenging task. Anyone can be busy. But who can truly relax?"[92] Over the next decade she would dwell on the effects of industriousness pounded into her—by her parents, we will learn, which is both telling and not at all surprising—but here this brief reflection is little more than a slight pause to the vicissitudes of an Asian American woman whose ambition to write matches that of the careers of our medical authors of the previous chapters and even our sick ones in this chapter.

On December 31, 2006, however, Lee wrote: "I am feeling strange. My brain is in a weird state right now—a combination of short brain games and lack of memory. While taking on the concept of a brain game earlier today, I suffered a memory overhaul. Now I can't say what I want to say or remember what I want to remember. It's just a weird situation."[93] She wished her readers a Happy New Year the following day, and then, on January 2, 2007, Lee composed a 472-word blog post titled "swimming ideas." Uncharacteristically, Lee doesn't use capital letters in the entry and describes her brain's actions as gustatory: "something in my brain burped. most of what i want to do is just out of my grasp. i feel like i know how to do them, but then when i go to do them, i just . . . CAN'T. day by day, i'm regaining my abilities, so i hope this is just temporary."[94] Later that day she tries to craft a whimsical post about herself, and then her blog goes silent for four days. On January 6, 2007, Lee gave her brain burp a name, a diagnosis: "Well. I totally had a stroke (seriously). The doctors are trying to figure out exactly why a 33 year old non-smoking woman would have a full blown stroke. I'll be back online when I can gather my thoughts, regain memories (I've lost some), etc. (I'm not talking about my initial attempts at gaining equilibrium, either). See you in a bit."[95]

From Blog to Memoir:
Christine Hyung-Oak Lee's Reassemblage

Over the course of the next few weeks, months, and years, Lee and her read-ers watched "Writing Under a Pseudonym" turn from a platform to catalog her writing process into an illness blog, one that would resemble Worrall's and Jennifer Ho's (and, to a certain extent, Fred Ho's Myspace entries and even Broyard's and Lorde's journal notes). Yet it became unwittingly a blog about writing not so much about illness as writing through illness. The blog would become an online version of what Lee would later call her "memory book," a journal that she kept after her stroke, during her convalescence. This journal and the blog would culminate on February 14, 2017, in the release of her memoir *Tell Me Everything You Don't Remember: The Stroke That Changed My Life.* The most immediate change to her life was the loss of short-term memory: severely damaged by a blood clot that prevented oxygen from reaching it, the dead tissue of her left thalamus left Lee unable to remember anything beyond fifteen-minute increments. Or, as she put it, "Without my thalamus, my brain went offline. It retained nothing."[96] This gives both her journal and her blog a primary, primal significance, a narrative surrogate for her lost memory: "My journal would act as my short-term memory bank, it turned out, for a long while to come."[97] Her journal and blog recorded in real time the manner in which her stroke interrupted the trajectory of her life narrative on December 31, 2006, and in the ensuing days profoundly and inexorably *disrupted* the ways that she had told her story, one that she could no longer resume. The blog becomes a testament to the narrative wreckage that Lee's illness wrought.

The blog also serves as the repository for Lee's reconstruction, a recalibra-tion through which the damage of the illness reveals, through its disruptive capacity, the emergence of a transformed self. The event of the stroke is a signal crisis for Lee that, in turn, prompts her to look anew at the story she had told herself and lived into until that event. In the ensuing days of chaos, which she describes as both uncontrollable anger and grief, Lee tills this material to coax metaphor out of her bodily and later existential crisis. The proximal cause of her stroke was patent foramen ovale (PFO), a gap between the left and right atria of the heart that fails to close after birth, which al-lowed a blood clot to bypass the lungs and work its way to Lee's brain. "For thirty-three years I had hole in my heart, and I did not know it," Lee writes to open her memoir. "There was an actual hole in my heart, an undiagnosed birth defect, with which I lived."[98] Yet this is not simply a colloquial descrip-tion of her PFO but a figuration of the narrative that she lived and what caused this narrative to end by way of her stroke: "And then there was the hole in my heart that I tried to dam up with other people's needs and then filled with resentment."[99] The narrative that Lee so painstakingly constructed before her stroke, she will discover, had at its core this "hole," a symptomatic lack from which emerges, she will learn, an accretion of dysfunction whose exposure is made possible by the stroke caused by the self-same hole. "There was a hole in my heart that made it impossible for me to be whole," she writes, "and then I had a stroke."[100] The stroke that changes Lee's life is the signal crisis that augurs the possibility of wholeness that her prior semblance of health made impossible.

There is no better expression of the fantasy of health and able-bodiedness than the value of industriousness pounded into her, as Lee alludes to in her opening blog entry. And the memoir slowly unpeels the toxicity of such values imposed on her, which, in turn, would become the precondition to her loss of voice and "wholeness." The literal hole in her heart, her PFO, makes it terribly difficult for Lee to breathe normally, a congenital condition that plagues her throughout her life and that she learns, Foucault-like, to endure and turn into a value of fortitude. It is, of course, a value reinforced by her immigrant parents, who raised her "to be tough and impervious to pain."[101] Lee recalls that her father "valued stoicism in the face of pain and strength at all costs." He refused medical care for a perforated small intestine, even though the ensuing sepsis sent him to extreme pain and life-threatening illness that resulted in doctors removing two feet of damaged intestinal tract. "He still brags about toughing it out," quips Lee.[102] From this she develops what Frank calls a dominating relation to her body to the point of trying to suppress her body's needs: depriving it of food, cutting it physically to mitigate deeper psychic wounds, manifesting an overall revulsion to it, a kind of hyper-Cartesian dualism. Lee writes, "The brain will excel in school. The brain will be the star. The mind will make up stories for the body's deficits. The mind will say her body is a failure. The mind will favor the brain."[103] Thus coterminous with the denigration of her body is Lee's favoring of the mind of her brain, that which Asian Americans, at the insistence of their parents, use to secure their futures of model minority success. While it is her parents—and in particular, her father—who erect the scaffold of this dysfunctional dualism, it is Lee who lives her life to perfect this narrative of success spurred on by the simultaneous elevation of her brain's mind and disavowal of her ostensibly uncontrollable body.

Lee's obsession with discipline and domination—of her mind and its regime over her body—informs the story that she tells about herself and the story she uses to live her life until her stroke. It is, in fact, this desire for

discipline that, Lee will later realize, constituted the very structures that allowed her to believe that this was her desire rather than the desire of others
around her. In a discussion about the distinction between semantic and episodic memory, Lee offers a litany of examples of past experiences that shaped
the inertia of her life's momentum: "Episodic memory is about the Sundays
my family spent hiking the San Gabriel Mountains, how I kept gasping for
air, and how no matter how often we went, I never found it easier."[104] This
remembrance of signs of her PFO, which as her younger self she ascribed to
pain endurance, her father's grit, then triggers other episodes of her voice
made lost: "I crumpled under my parents' wishes for me to become a doctor. . . . [T]hey thought a writing career was too daring."[105] Likewise, Lee's
marriage to Adam, which she initially regards as an assertion of agency and
revolt against her Korean immigrant parents (he is Jewish, and they elope),
becomes yet another instance of the loss of her "voice." After recounting that
Adam would not assent to a do-not-resuscitate order if she were incapacitated,
insisting that the decision was his, Lee reflects on living indefinitely on life
support as a "kind of death": "In a sense, I was already not living my own
life. I thought I was, because I had a career and I paid my own bills. But I
was living Adam's life, cheerleading him and not myself."[106] The irony of her
obsession for discipline, then, is that it served only to deepen her subjection
to social narrative frames that circumscribed the desires of others as her own,
a relegation of duty as her sole form of desire. "The thing is, I'd lost my voice
in so many ways already, before the stroke even occurred," she writes. "I had
been unable to say, I am trapped in my life. That my obligations were inter-
fering with my personal dreams. I made up rules and stuck to them because
that was safe. It was, however, not brave."[107]

You'll notice in the previous paragraph that the passages from the memoir work their way backward. Lee acknowledges her lost voice early in the
memoir. The day of her stroke represents not so much a critical event in her
life as a critical and radical reordering of narrative, a story in which linear
form will no longer hold. The days and months that would follow brought
about what is so often the case in illness: a crisis in an identity when restitution is no longer available, a self bereft of a progressive narrative of restoration, a self thrown into chaos. All that she valued of herself, which included
a photographic memory that would allow her to quote passages from books
or recall credit card numbers of men who bought her drinks, is inaccessible
to Lee, the damage to her brain disordering the very architecture of her life:
"The stroke pushed on the weakest and most untested seams of my psyche.
Where before I could never feel vulnerable—I wouldn't let myself—I was
now vulnerable all the time. Where before I could not ask for help, I needed

to ask for assistance to get through the day. Where before I could not allow myself to feel sad, I lost the ability to dam up my emotions. Where before I always planned in the interest of being in control, it was now impossible to do so. A part of myself really had died."[108] The stroke has Lee peer into a looking glass, where she discovers a self that is the converse of her formerly able-bodied version. And the death of this former self—which, she will discern, is truly gone, even after she "recovers" from her stroke—will send her into a deeper chaos from which she almost doesn't emerge: "Later in my recovery, when I was well enough to understand what had happened to me, to realize my deficits and become depressed about my stalled progress, when I wondered if my old life would ever return in any familiar form, I pondered taking a big dose of warfarin and then slicing my wrists."[109] The discovery of a new self as a former one dies, together with a desire to end this self by suicide, highlights the peril of the crisis born of the chaos that arrives in the wake of Lee's stroke, the double-edgedness of chaos that can never be mitigated or qualified: "Chaos stories show how quickly the props that other stories depend on can be kicked away. The limitation is that chaos is no way to live."[110] Gone are fantasies of progress, of linearity itself. For a time, Lee recalls, she can exist only in an interregnum.

What approximates this terrifying and liminal state is Lee's resonance with the two protagonists in *Slaughterhouse-Five*, Kurt Vonnegut's classic novel about war, and more important for our sake, trauma. The novel first comes to materialize her loss of short-term memory, on which she prided herself deeply, as Lee cannot move beyond the first paragraph of the novel, let alone the first page: "I started reading it right before my stroke, and I continued to read it in the days following. But I was reading the same page, over and over. The first page. The first paragraph. I did not know this until later."[111] This first paragraph, which begins with the sentence, "All this happened, more or less," is told from the vantage of Vonnegut, the narrator and author who confirms the historical (and autobiographical) foundations of the novel: his terrible and traumatic experience in World War II and, in particular, his witnessing of the Allied bombing of Dresden. In Lee's memoir, the "more or less" that also happens is the catastrophe of her stroke, how it inflicts on Lee the narrative-shattering trauma that Vonnegut shapes through his novel and that his protagonist character Billy Pilgrim experiences. Lee will read this passage over and over, recapitulating the narrator's words without remembering them, which disrupts and replaces the normative reading practice with a static, traumatic one. She can't get past the event; the event overtakes her sense of narrative.

Thus, Lee, like Billy Pilgrim, coincidentally, serendipitously becomes "unstuck in time" and engages in her own sort of time travel, just as Vonnegut's novel's protagonist hurtles through time. "Like Billy Pilgrim in *Slaughterhouse-Five*," Lee analogizes, "I experienced my life like a random series of moments without beginning or end. All points in time existed simultaneously—and for me, that was in the present moment. Nothing happened before, because I could not recall the past, and nothing happened after, because I could not comprehend the future."[112] Following Vonnegut's style, Lee's memoir sets out a narrative that is both randomly and deliberatively recursive. The passage that precedes her explicit comparison to Pilgrim has Lee narrating mundane actions that are direct and simple, yet disjointed and arbitrary; the actions and sentences form no broader coherent meaning: "I brushed my teeth. I petted my dog. And then I sat. I sat for hours. Or maybe minutes. I was unstuck in time."[113] Such experience of disjointedness, in which her sense of order is barely kept together by the simplest of syntax, then has Lee hurtle backward in time to her birth and her upbringing in Southern California, through college, and up to her marriage to Adam, an exercise in semantic memory, as if she is willing herself into a form of linear progress that brain and body refuse. Like Pilgrim's, Lee's time travels are signal reminders of the trauma of the stroke and its irrevocable impact on narrative temporality: the linearity of restitution gone, Lee must learn to craft a narrative in which trauma and woundedness are constitutive elements. Like Vonnegut, Lee will utter multiple times "and so on" and "so it goes"; in *Slaughterhouse-Five*, these phrases are verbal mitigations, tic-like, of the precarity of life and the arbitrariness of death in warfare (and, by extension, in civilian life). In *Tell Me Everything*, these phrases point to the contingency of the body: Lee exerts every effort to become herself through the model minority expectations of her parents and, later, her Jewish husband, Adam, and his family, a life drive that results in a stroke, her body betraying her social desire: "So it goes."

Lee began her blog to document the undertaking of her novel and was interrupted inexorably by the stroke. The blog and, in turn, the memoir then turns writing into an altogether different vocation, less an index to her ambition that would match the economic or cultural capital of Adam than a mode of reenchanting her life, writing as a movement for and beyond survival and toward a flourishing with and through her trauma. "Writing saved my life," she writes definitely. "I did not write that down [in my memory book]. But of that I am certain."[114] The soteriology of writing, however, is not recovery but reconstruction. Lee never returns to a semblance of her pre-stroke self but must build, in the aftermath of chaos and trauma, an illness-borne afterlife. "It took me years to be ready to write about my stroke," Lee recalls late in her memoir. "I did try to write about it. I wanted to write about it. I attempted to write an essay about my stroke no fewer than eleven times—there was no narrative, there was no structure to it. I wasn't ready. All in all, it took eight years to write it down. It took that long because I tried for eight years to put the stroke behind me. It wasn't until I had a baby and I had postpartum depression and my husband of fifteen years left me that I could look at the stroke."[115] Lee's stroke is so disruptive that it leaves next to nothing of her former life from which she can build her post-stroke story, the elements of her pre-stroke life a rubble that precipitates deeper crisis, a depression, and a loss of her familial and conjugal structures. She has, as she puts it, "no narrative, no structure" to the stroke and no narrative or structure to what follows, at least initially. So writing becomes a means to reconstruct a new syntax of her life, a reordering of her neurology and of what constitutes what Lee might consider her good.

Arthur Frank notes that this recursive journey that the illness story tells, shorn of the illusion of restitution and struggling to emerge out of chaos, mandates this different, oblique relation to how the body remembers itself: "This self is not so newly discovered as newly connected to its own memory."[116] In deep contrast to how Lee related to herself prior to the stroke, this new connection that she forges with her memory is not simply a return of her mind, but a renewed partnership with her body, still wounded, that she had long disavowed because she believed it failed to live up to the model minority expectation that she demanded of it and her mind: "But my mind and body, long at war with each other, would come to a great peace beyond my imagination. . . . My mind realized it needed my body, needed to recognize its new and strange strength."[117] Indeed, she commits to end the long tyranny of her mind over her body, one that plagued her with eating disorders, self-mutilation, and, at times, sex with others "to run away from my pain." "Now it was my body's turn to lead," Lee resolves. "I began to listen to my body, instead of ignoring its needs."[118] This, too, is the vocation of writing her stroke, writing as a material effect of the self narrating her trauma not as escape but as reckoning, a witness to the body that broke and must be seen for Lee's new narrative to emerge. Or, as Frank might put it, "The witness of suffering must be seen as a whole body, because embodiment is the essence of witness."[119]

It is the stroke, the catalyzing and cauterizing wound, that teaches Lee "lessons, many of which revolved around writing." In fact, she suggests, it is the loss of her ability to write that enables her to understand the very nature of writing and her relationship to it, the complex interplay between memory and language, neurology and imagination: "I learned that memory comes in modules. That narrative comprises pieces that must be woven together to create a unique texture and pattern. They are connected by pieces of thread."[120] Note both the artisanry imbedded in Lee's metaphors of textile, figures that are as idiosyncratic as they are fragile: her memory woven into narrative, hanging by thread. In place of the steely endurance she learned from her father as a means of maneuvering, Lee finds that her writing after her stroke brings her into raw, open emotion, a discovery of language that was heretofore unavailable to her. And with this comes a realization of the vocation of the writer herself. At a workshop led by the novelist Chris Abani, Lee hesitates to share from Abani's assignment, which is to write a deeply personal anecdote. After a long pause, Abani asks, "Then why are you a writer?" Lee has no answer and then describes Abani's understanding of the writer's vocation: "He said that a writer cannot be private like that. We must share our truths. We must be brave."[121] She continues, "And so I agreed," then offers a description of this kernel of the memoir, this decision to write about what she calls her "year of grief." Writing is the means through which Lee's vulnerable body can also be communicative and dyadic, not simply wounded to itself but allowing her wounds to resonate with the tender organs of readers, the cultivation of an altogether different community of other wounded storytellers, whether they are writers or not. "The language of my stroke is forever in my brain," Lee recalls, and it is this language that serves as the alphabet to narrate a new kind of citizenship she carries in her sojourn in the land where model minorities and the able-bodied still roam, if only a bit longer. [122] It is a language that moves more slowly and more messily, but one that calls Lee and the other Asian American wounded storytellers to imagine a community that bears the mark of particular, respective, and shared pain, and one that is simultaneously, and counterintuitively, Asian American. It may very well be the witness of the marginal, the barely visible but always noticed, Asian American body made vulnerable though illness, disability, or other kinds of catastrophe that will provide the basis of some insight, of what might happen, what is possible when the model minority is finally done in—one hopes sooner, but inevitably later.

Conclusion: Whither Asian American Afterlives?

Which leads me back to Paul Kalanithi and Julie Yip-Williams and this desire to redeem their ends not just as "good" deaths but as reminders of the afterlife of model minorities after they are gone. Because they could not complete their memoirs, their partners, Lucy Kalanithi and Joshua Williams, respectively, wrote epilogues that chronicle their dying moments, bringing readers to their bedside as they breathe their last, as the title of both memoirs suggest: breath becoming air, the miracle (of life) unwinding. Stylistically, they differ in approach. While Lucy Kalanithi writes in exquisite detail about Paul's rather sudden final days and hours of life, during which we watch him, Lucy, and the greater family all express their goodbyes verbally and somatically—"With my heart breaking, I climbed into the last bed we would share"—Joshua Williams describes more generically that Julie died with family and friends surrounding her, as if to keep readers a room away from her final moments. But both epilogues recast the illness memoir into a contemporary *Ars moriendi*, a narrative meditation on Paul and Julie "dying well," less because they offered examples of ideal ways of dying than, perhaps, because these short reflections by the spouses of these ill Asian Americans must account for and bear witness to the fact of declension as the end of even the model minority story, every model minority story. "How can I die? How can I be dying?" Joshua recounts Julie asking aloud in an opioid-induced fog state during her last days, long after treatment bore no curative hope. Yet these incredulous questions also contain within them the insight of Asian American ill pedagogy that nudges readers beyond a model minority algorithm of squeezing optimal success out of struggle and suffering. Instead, the partners seek to read in the truncated fetch of their now dead loved ones a differential value added to Asian American life, one that can only be understood in sickness and death. As Lucy Kalanithi writes, "The earth is quickly turned over by worms, the processes of nature marching on, reminding me of what Paul saw and what I now carry deep in my bones, too: the inextricability of life and death, and the ability to cope, to find meaning despite this, because of this. What happened to Paul was tragic, but he was not a tragedy."[123] Joshua Williams figures his narrative memorial as a way to make Julie's question—How can I die?—one that points to a different rule of life from the one expected of Asian Americans: "It is in the acceptance of truth [of illness and death] that real living begins. Conversely, avoidance of truth is the denial of life."[124] It may be a coincidence that both authors of these Asian American memoirs' epilogues are white, but it is no less significant, as if, finally, white America can let go of its fantasy of and for Asian Americans and their expected racial form so that maybe Asian America might someday disbelieve this article of faith and live inside a different mythos. Other things would still need to happen, for sure. But maybe, in working from the ends of Asian America, there is a means to start this project, again, for the first time.

Illness as Method

I think being a literary critic is highly carcinogenic.
Have there been any studies?

—Anatole Broyard

Sympathy for a Germ? A Scholar's Account

Like many illness memoirs, Patrick Anderson's autoethnography, *Autobiography of a Disease*, describes the moment he moves from experiencing and embodying his illness—a severe infection by methicillin-resistant Staphylococcus aureus (MRSA) bacteria—toward illness's representation through narrative. Returning to the hospital after initial optimism by medical staff that intravenous and oral antibiotics would eradicate the strain gives way to a starker reality, and Anderson prepares for what will be a long and terrifying flight of medicalization, pain, indignity, several major surgeries, and, eventually, a reparative relation to his body by asking his mother for a paper and pen. This would be the first time he'd engaged in any writing since his illness, save for the medical forms that he filled out and signed upon admission to and discharge from the hospital. "He wrote for several minutes without ceasing," goes the narrative to describe Anderson's activity, achingly slow but steady. "'So broken, so many parts of me. Finally feels like there's a plan to put me back together again. First time in ages I've felt like I might have an *after* to this, an after to live in and fill out' was the opening bit."[1] In his first act of writing, Anderson composes two truths about himself and about illness, not as anomaly but as ontological condition: first, illness breaks him, shatters him so that his reconstruction mandates a "plan"; second, and relatedly, this shattering of his former healthy self signifies a death of sorts, his life after illness "an after to live in and fill out," or, as he will call it later, an "afterlife of illness." Of course, in the moment of this writing, all remains contingent: the "after" is not at all a guarantee, and only a few pages later we will, with Anderson, realize how close he was to not getting to have this afterlife, how close we were to never being able to read this story, his afterlife an obituary rather than a memoir.

I say "this story" and not his story because, as Anderson emphatically puts it in his foreword to the book, while "this book is about illness," it is also "about how we make sense of being ill."[2] And Anderson opts from the outset to decenter "Patrick" in this experience, to turn the MRSA bacteria that plagued and pained him into the protagonist, with Patrick stepping in as principal interlocutor but not the only one. MRSA is chiefly responsible for shattering Anderson's world, but others also bear this burden and weight of reckoning, which include the health-care staff tasked with destroying the infection to save Patrick's life, even at the expense of his suffering, Patrick's biological and chosen family, and Anderson himself. "This book, then," Anderson reflects, "understands illness not as a patient's monologue or biography, but as a profoundly social, richly durational, and multiply perspectival encounter. It seeks to describe how illness makes meaning of the world even as it threatens to dissemble the world in which it occurs."[3] Note here how much more capacious Anderson's depiction of his illness is, his relationship to the disease that ails him almost on the verge of affection, in sharp contrast to the war rhetoric Fred Ho and even Audre Lorde might employ to narrate their relationship to their respective cancers. The deep sociality that Anderson hopes to narrate acknowledges both the chaos of illness and the potential for new forms of relation, meaning, and value to come from the woundedness borne by the ill person. Insofar as Anderson's narrative is constituted by a fictionalized narration of MRSA, the story of his illness reveals little malice or ill intent. Notwithstanding its status as the principal micro-bugaboo in hospitals across the United States, MRSA's desire to coexist and live with Patrick and other human hosts is couched in terms of interdependence and even necessity. As MRSA narrates early in Anderson's book, *"After a while, we realized that we were exactly what [Patrick] needed, an insurrection in the deadening habits of daily life, a wake-up to his own vulnerability. We held our ground for his benefit as much as our own."*[4] Anderson shares a proximity with MRSA that is fraught, even deadly, even as it is also symbiotic and pedagogical. MRSA desires to live just as Anderson does. This mutually constituted survival instinct makes MRSA both disruptive and generative—or, perhaps more accurate, generative because disruptive—to Anderson's reconstruction of himself as a person whose embodiment, now pent up with new social forms interacting with his body, must accede to new demands of representation. At the very least, there is more than grudging respect in MRSA's subaltern resistance; it is Anderson, then, who chooses to narrate them as worthy of representation.

This distribution of agency, care, and suffering across multiple subjectivities for what is otherwise a deeply intimate narrative about his illness—at one point a doctor kisses Anderson on the forehead, which leaves him, he writes, "feeling suddenly quite warm—but simultaneously completely broken"[5]—stems, of course, from his interdisciplinary training in anthropology, performance, and cultural studies. The almost instinctual reflex to scribe field notes as soon as he is conscious and (barely) able is matched by the scholarly disposition that circumscribes Anderson's narrative, which allows him to engage and assess critically the very work of his narration. This isn't to say that those without doctoral training in ethnography can't accomplish such a vantage; it is simply to note that, for better or worse, Anderson's predilection for reflective thick description of social worlds leads him to what looks, from the perspective of memoir, radically experimental. To a scholar, especially of anthropology, Anderson's "autobiography" is a very well-composed and well-written scholarly monograph. The critical, even fundamental, questions that anchor the book's argument and method—if a person's illness can have either—come at the end, as if to remind the reader that the intimacy of Anderson's ill story is also an ethnographic stratum through which he builds a general ecology of illness. "If illness is a *social* rather than strictly individual phenomenon," Anderson poses in the afterword, "how might narrative negotiate the *distribution* of *agency*—to caregivers, surgeons, lab workers, pharmacists, and others—alongside its obligations to honor and maintain the *specificity* of the experience of being-ill? If narrative is human invention, how might *objects' and non-sentient* beings' ways-of-knowing be *translated* and *valued* as *equally informative, equally important, even equally aesthetic representations?*"[6] I gesture emphatically to the terms italicized in the quotation to highlight the observational skills that contemporary humanities scholars, social scientists, and cultural studies practitioners are trained to do well, which is to *pay attention* to the social worlds that constitute a subjectivity, however hidden, however differentiated other subjectivities might be from your own, and see how their relation builds a deeply imbricated, complicated, and meaningful story barely contained by a phrase such as "my illness." This isn't to make little or light of Anderson's critical capacities. To the contrary, *Autobiography of a Disease* demonstrates the extent to which a queer/disability studies analytic can reveal a range of affective and material dimensions to illness beyond the obviously and increasingly limited scope of the "physician-patient relationship." It is one that isn't impossible for someone not trained as Anderson is, but as one can see upon reading the book, such training surely helps.

This chapter then wonders explicitly what is revealed about illness when it finds itself represented in the mode of writing that a tiny demography of the United States is trained professionally to write—the scholarly mono-graph—a genre as constitutive to the contemporary academy as it is (often) laconic to those who don't traffic in the currency of its cultural capital. This chapter thus risks considerably having an "inside-the-beltway" feel, but I think this endeavor is worth making for this very simple reason: scholars, their ostensible and fantasized life of the mind notwithstanding, get sick and die, too. And if the vocation of the scholar of culture and society, whether she examines through books or film, community meeting or street corner, or spoken word event or library archive or museum exhibit, is to unearth and exhume the range of possibility of human (and, yes, nonhuman) life and give it some understanding or social meaning, then the experience of illness, even one's own, is archive or data set or plentiful text enough. Illness deserves as much attention to the editorial, methodological, and hermeneutic expecta-tions and rigors as any other primary source, subjected to and illuminated by the critical inquiry of good scholarship. Yet like Anderson, I want to make the case that illness (or disability or, more generally, woundedness) constitutes an existential mode for the scholar that exceeds a totalizing epistemological cap-ture, as "the constant stream of disorientation, misrecognition, and radical undoing . . . occupies the very heart of illness's ontology," illness as instigating "crises that push the limits of knowing and knowability."[7]

Illness then works in tension with the scholar's impulse for comprehen-siveness and rigor, even as any scholarly book must circumscribe and ac-knowledge that certain things are *beyond the scope of one's argument.* Such a phrase is often composed with a tinge of regret, as if the argument's scope falls short of the intellectual desire to know more and make it comprehen-sible: thus, Anderson's compulsion to write even as he is contorted in waves of pain. Still, as I've been saying throughout this book, *pace* Arthur Frank, illness interrupts and can do so without ceasing. Thus, it becomes an event horizon for the very warrant of the scholarly enterprise, as we shall see not only in Anderson but in the other scholars to whom I'll pay attention here. More than thirty years ago, Elaine Scarry characterized bodily pain as the hub whose radiation "unmade" the world and, specifically, the language we use to then "make" the world.[8] She, of course, focused her attention on two structures of pain, torture and war, modes that have been taken up to de-scribe the experience of illness and its medical treatment. For Scarry, the body in pain was isolated from others, a form of alienation through which the subject's world could be overtaken and overwhelmed by the inflictor of pain. The body in pain is made passive; likewise, the ill scholar finds herself undone by the disruption of illness, the world she is tasked to explain with critical insight a distance away and removed. What method can attend to illness's interruption? What discipline can cordon the body undone?

Living in Differential Prognosis: S. Lochlann Jain

There is in Anderson's account, amid his chaos, disorientation, and radical undoing, a moment that we might call epiphanic—or, at least, an instance of deliberate agency on his part with regard to the medical treatment of his illness. After returning to the hospital, Anderson is told by Dr. Shin that the infection has spread so deeply into his hip bone that the original surgery that he had planned will not work. Dr. Shin will therefore discharge him until a bed in a new hospital better suited to Anderson's grave condition can be found. "Tell you what. I've got a different plan. I refuse," Anderson responds, disallowing the hospital's release from liability, insisting on staying in the hospital, demanding further care. His refusal to move is initially an affront to Dr. Shin but a rallying cry to Anderson's advocates—his mother, the nursing staff, even his primary care physician, who describes Anderson's confrontation with Dr. Shin as "remarkable"—to be ever more emboldened to insist on care on his terms, not just the physician's and surgeon's. While he doesn't dwell on it, Anderson subtly hints at the racial and gendered privilege he wields both invisibly and effortlessly against his Asian American doctor, an instance of what contemporary medicine might call "patient-centered care" that is largely unavailable to people differently raced or gendered. The very next chapter has Anderson narrating a fictionalized account of his Black nurse, Sheila, walking along the streets of Oakland. After witnessing a white man's assertion for his own care, she reflects on the lack of care afforded to her son, whose belated diagnosis of meningitis would kill him, and whose physician's response was little more than paternalistic and benignly neglectful: "Should have brought him sooner."[9] It is an asymmetry of affective and material resources that isn't lost on Anderson, as he later reflects on those who drown under the tsunami of medical bills and cannot rely on a mother or friends such as his for support.[10] Despite his initial shock, Dr. Shin listens to Anderson and finds him a hospital room right away. Likewise, and later, Anderson doesn't need to file for bankruptcy, as the hospital waives his medical bills after his mother, Deirdre, helps clear them.

At the time of his illness, Anderson was a graduate student at Berkeley, so he was actually quite poor, but people still listened to him, thanks to his extensive and intimate network of family and friends, as well as to the network of unconscious bias that made his voice—uttered by a queer white man, however constrained by illness and suffering—still heard. Such was not the case, at least initially, for Asian American scholars who have written about their experiences of illness. Take, for instance, S. Lochlann Jain, who suffuses their book *Malignant*, about the ubiquity of cancer in the United States, with anecdotes of their breast cancer. Their story, however, begins with disbelief: Jain's initial oncologist flatly refuses to believe that the lump on their breast might be cancerous and, even after the threat of a second opinion, opts for a fine needle aspiration, a procedure that results in far more false negatives than core biopsies. Jain wonders what accounts for their doctor, whom they call Dr. Nordic, to underpin her peak whiteness, to categorically *not* listen to her patient: "Wasn't I friendly enough? Did she think of me as a whiny patient who should just go away? Or maybe I wasn't insistent enough. Was the dismissal because of my dark complexion (race) or my sexuality? Did she just think I was too young to get cancer?"[11] Jain's ruminations seem initially to settle on ageism on the part of Dr. Nordic, as they then cite examples of other young adults (under forty) whose misdiagnoses led some of them to suffer terminal metastases of their cancers. Their personal stories become part of their larger ethnography, or as Jain puts it, "My patient self meets my anthropologist's self here, drifting downstream with the alligators. I've collected stories of young adults' delayed diagnoses for a purpose beyond just some weird form of self-consolation," a scholarly intuition that "something bigger is going on."[12]

This something bigger is the laconic phenomenon we think we know when we say "cancer." "Cancer," Jain writes, "in all its nounishness refers to everything . . . and nothing. . . . What on earth, then, do we mean when we refer to this concept, cancer?"[13] Despite biomedical efforts to cast an optimistic glean on the history of the cancer, as Siddhartha Mukherjee is at pains to do in his "biography of cancer" *The Emperor of All Maladies*, as a slow but progressive journey of "beating" this variegated disease, the consuming experience of cancer in contemporary social life means that it cannot be compartmentalized, quarantined like infectious diseases that have since come under control through vaccination and antibiotics.[14] Jain argues that cancer refuses any objective measure; instead, it is "better understood as a set of relationships—economic, sentimental, medical, personal, ethical, institutional, statistical. . . . not as a disease awaiting a cure, but as a constitutive aspect of American social life, economics, and science. *Malignant* builds on this idea, presenting cancer as a process and as a social field, while also exploring *its brutal effects at the level of individual experience*."[15] In this last sentence we see Jain's anthropological training kicking in: to examine cancer as a process and social field, it becomes subject to the rigors of discursive analysis, as it might by any good Foucauldian or disability studies theorist, the valuations of human embodiment socially constructed and constituted; to pay attention to individuals is to grant them Bourdieuian agency, some meaning there even in suffering.

The task of discerning the interests that determine "how and when cancer is named" and "the interests that produce and treat the disease," and thereby "unraveling the guiding logics of these institutions," are compelling features of Jain's book, which demonstrate how their meticulous research and critical vantage make the most of methodological exposure.[16] In trying to uncover the reasons for their doctor's misdiagnosis and casual dismissal of their concerns, Jain explores the complexity of medical malpractice and liability law and notes that, while not fully antagonistic toward patients subject to physician error, the legal system's structural indeterminacy cannot overcome a fundamental paradox in the law: physicians make mistakes in diagnosis and treatment, yet the expectation of causality (i.e., the doctor's mistake caused my husband to die) is so difficult to establish that the law "serves to strengthen the aura of cancer as a quasi-mystical, ungraspable cultural and biological phenomenon."[17] What's more, physicians are not incentivized to announce the mistakes of colleagues under oath. Jain offers a stinging critique of Atul Gawande's book *Complications: A Surgeon's Notes on an Imperfect Science*, ostensibly written to "humanize" doctors by showcasing their fallibilities while ultimately arguing that techniques, checklists, and peer oversight aim to make medical practice "more" perfect, however impossible that goal is.[18] They see past Gawande's rhetorical attempts at medical humility that mask more fundamental mistakes of an existential order:

> Gawande mistakes the individual surgeon who has to learn and who will make mistakes throughout his career for someone who should be responsible for those mistakes only to the profession (and not to the patient). He further confuses the compensatory function of law for a moral system of blame—a pervasive condition in medical professional culture. . . . [H]e ignores the questions of patient knowledge of error or whether patients being practiced on should pay reduced rates for care. . . . Aiming for perfection is certainly an admirable goal, but structural challenges render it impossible.[19]

Gawande's medical liberalism cannot fully adjudicate the misplaced structures of accountability and responsibility, which reinforce rather than mitigate the asymmetries of power that exist between those performing medical practice and those subjected to those practices, even at the level of civil and criminal law, nominally outside biomedical control.

Jain is equally trenchant in their examination of the "gold standard of evidentiary medicine, the randomized controlled trial (RCT)," in which people in one group may receive an experimental treatment while another receives either a placebo or standard treatment.[20] The RCT's seeming scientific objectivity to determine the efficacy of an emergent treatment obscures what Jain calls the "thanatopolitics" of this method. While recounting the story of a late-stage cancer drug in the midst of research trials in which a researcher notes that more than a thousand (1,050) people would need to relapse in order to collect data, Jain points to the perverse temporality of this particular RCT: "There *will be* 1,050 recurrences, indeed, . . . there *must be*, and . . . these recurrences will occur in both the treatment and nontreatment groups."[21] The promise of progressive medicine through statistical data of RCT belies its horrific side effect: "The RCT erases the very human subjects that enabled its possibility, legitimating its dead through the promise of a future cure."[22] The RCT relies on what Jain calls the "mortality effect," a statistical methodology in which medical futurity relies on the ever present fresh dead who are the mortal evidence that a new treatment renews the promise of medical cure, a promise reserved chiefly, if at all, for a later generation, long after the casualties of the trial are buried. In this sense, the RCT, Jain argues, is the methodology of biomedical power par excellence: "Suffering and death undergird a system that works differently for different participants, constructing some members as experts and others as dependents. Stating the paradox of the mortality effect this baldly enables us to see how the RCT creates a temporal hierarchy in which the mortality of some props up, or allows, the immortality of others. This mortality effect, however necessary, intensifies the hierarchies of medicine."[23] Cancer and the war against it thus drive a political economy whose currency traffics not only in wide circulation of monetary but also human capital. Medicine needs its bodies to promise others their cure.

But while we may shake our heads in outrage at cancer's political economy, it is "*its brutal effects at the level of individual experience*" that leave us bereft in silent horror. The suffering born of misdiagnosis and of wondering what side of the RCT lottery one is on are not abstract imaginings but instances that Jain themself experienced. Their study of cancer's everythingness and nothingness does not discount but, in fact, highlights the necessity of insisting on honoring the individuality of this experience even in—especially in—its pervasiveness. So alongside their critique of cancer's economic and institutional structures, Jain inhabits the lives of those stricken with the disease, in first-person memoiristic accounts, in retreats with those in remission and those whose cancer has recurred, and perhaps most important, to turn their own experience with breast cancer into important scholarly data. "It would be easier to play the role of the detached guide," Jain admits, but they lean into their cancer because in the affective experience of cancer's politics, individuation matters: "We need to delve into cancer discussions that we'd rather hide from. And so, after looking long and hard from the canoe for seven years, I've leapt into the white water. I invite my readers to explore with me the very things we (read, a slightly lonely 'I') most want to shy away from."[24] These things that we'd rather hide from and shy away from are the collectively dreaded and individually felt terror of what Jain calls "living in prognosis," that affective state after a cancer diagnosis "that severs the idea of a timeline and all the usual ways we orient ourselves in time: age, generation, and stage of an assumed lifespan."[25] "Cancer and prognosis form oncology's double helix," the very heart of this medical specialization, but living in prognosis that is the ontological state of a person with cancer points also to the fact of the general condition of prognosis that is human life until it isn't: "We assume survival—until we don't. You don't really think about it until you are called into the position of survivorship (by age, illness, anxiety, prognosis), until you are asked in some way to inhabit the category, to live amid those who are not, in fact, surviving."[26] Jain's use of the second-person address here is a deliberate interpellation of the reader not as a detached, abstracted fellow theorist but, rather, as a similarly embodied person who is always already at risk of living the precarity of prognosis, even if you are, at this moment, as far you can tell, healthy, like Jain addressing a former self not yet aware of their diagnosis. Illnesses such as cancer can hail you, illuminate your individuality in ways unlike any other. It is as if Jain is saying this moment: reader, you might have cancer right now, as I did. How does it feel to be always already maybe ill and dying?

Jain recounts that when their doctor half-heartedly shared with them the diagnosis of their cancer, they "felt as though she turned me into a pitiable blister beetle." Such an event, they acknowledge, happens all the time, "more commonplace than a college education . . . yet, when it happens to us, how can it not be noteworthy?"[27] The absolutely ordinary because ubiquitous phenomenon of a cancer diagnosis, which is *also* an absolutely singular event of devastation, spurs the scholar to find in their experience something noteworthy, something as significant as a cultural text for a literary critic or a heretofore unregarded community for the anthropologist. For as a chronicle of a journey into Susan Sontag's kingdom of the sick, the academic monograph strives to wrest something approximating scholarly meaning out of the banality of illness whose treatment reduces them further to bare or sometimes posthuman life. It's perhaps for this reason that even those deeply critical of the academic memoir, of life writings by university scholars, balk when they confront the professor who is, because of illness or disability, unwell in some capacity.

In her monograph critically appraising the rise of the contemporary academic memoir, Cynthia Franklin identifies the genre as one that emergences principally as expressions in the wake of what she calls the crisis of legitimacy of the humanities as a field and the university as an institution, the academic memoir serving as a "barometer for the state of humanities during a period of crisis."[28] She attributes the rise also to the countervailing forces of the rise of the "academic star system" that vaulted a few into a kind of celebrity status, even as the promise of public-facing humanities scholars (and, arguably, scholarship) largely failed "to achieve hoped-for transformations in the public sphere."[29] To this extent, the life writing of the academic for public reading consumption is a symptom of the neoliberalizing individuation logic of the university that simultaneously underscores the "university's estrangement from a wider public"; writing a memoir can be a sign of retreat from a politics of engagement *or* an attempt to engage the public through a form that is already appealing to a nonacademic readership.

Inherent in the genre of the memoir, Franklin worries, is the seductive power of the story of the individual and, with it, the attendant ideologies of individualism, liberalism, and a conservative form of humanism that simultaneously obscures the forms of domination necessary for the cultivation of the individual as liberal subject. Mindful of such ideological embeddedness and investment, Franklin hopes for and foregrounds memoirs that deploy the personal voice to highlight such relations of power and ways that structure and institutional relations constitute the academic self. This mode of critique allows her then to illuminate those memoirs she identifies as exhibiting what she calls a "nonexclusionary humanism" that work against the genre's tendency to privilege a form of interiority that evacuates the political in favor of the taking up the genre to "communicate a political agenda or an institutional critique."[30] The ideal academic memoir, for Franklin, is a kind of life writing that does what we have come to expect of critical writing in the humanities—namely, a form of reading for exposure such as historicist/materialist or psychoanalytically symptomatic, or what Eve Kosofsky Sedgwick called paranoid reading.[31] Franklin's study must peer at this paradox: to read the stories of individual academics writing about themselves and evaluating the extent to which they write about others more than they write about themselves. To do so would be an idealized memoir that jettisons an unexamined individualism for life writing that can "make interventions in academic and wider cultural spheres that carry on the work of third world, feminist, disability, and cultural studies scholars and activists."[32]

While some individual memoirists buck and militate against the individualizing elements of memoir, and even in these special cases not unproblematically, the memoirs that engage with or express insights provided through disability and disability studies bear special status in Franklin's formulation. Because disability studies critically examines how the idealized individual is imagined through its disavowal of presumably less valued because disabled counterparts *and* redefines the terms of humanity and whose lives are worth living, the disability memoir can powerfully conjoin the individual's testimony as a way to engage with empathy with this subject *while* offering the "institutional analysis" that might deconstruct more narrow views of the human. In short, Franklin argues, the disability memoir opens up the "possibility of an expansive, inclusive humanism—one that can reinvigorate cultural theories and make a case in the wider culture for the humanities' value as a carrier of human rights."[33]

It is at this moment, when she advances the prospect of disability's capacity toward an inclusive humanism that moves beyond the analytically feeble individualistic, that she inserts the personal. This intimate and, yes, individual relation to disability and illness gives Franklin an insight that then enchants the form of writing disability memoir. This moment becomes Franklin's own disability memoir, an opportunity to inhabit the very expansive humanism that she hopes for in her readings of others:

> While I was writing this chapter my work was punctuated—and at times brought to a standstill—by a series of crises involving illness and disability. Several family members, friends, and colleagues experienced severe depressions and other critical illnesses. In addition, I spent many telephone hours with friends on leaves of absence to care for terminally ill parents. Entering an illness or disability—one's own or a loved one's—is, as any number of disability studies critics have attested, to enter an alternate often isolated world, at the same time as such an experience is absolutely ordinary, and to be expected as people age.[34]

These personal encounters then compelled Franklin to reassess her critical appraisal of memoirs that she considered conscious of their privilege, whether because of gender, race, class, or tenure status. Undone by a loved one's severe mental illness, she felt in that moment an "utter unimportance of my own academic position, and by a sudden and foreboding sense that I had seriously underestimated the importance of the feelings expressed by those academics I was subjecting to critique."[35] While she remains resolute in her argument—after all, her book rests on it—Franklin's own autobiographical story in this critical consideration of memoir illuminates an ambiguity that exceeds the rhetorical expectations of argument, as often life's vulnerability does so well, in caring not one bit about one's hermeneutic horizons.

This is the paradox of taking seriously the singular in illness. Illness (and disability) simultaneously isolates and situates you in a system or web of relations, more often than not with the ill or disabled person at the whim of others whose differential subjectivities allow them to pass you by. And it makes things that heretofore had been hidden from you—or, sometimes more accurately, what you actively didn't want to notice—shimmer with such intensity that the surrounding environment vibrates with electric relation. For Franklin, the argument against liberal individualism couldn't stop her individuation in the face of illness, disability, and death; instead, "Such experiences have brought home to me what my arguments diminish—as they also have underlined the importance of empathy, and the fact that to a certain extent empathy is situation-specific and learned."[36] Illness is a condition of vulnerability and an end to the fiction of autonomy, an opening to a pedagogy of interdependency if one allows empathy—or some other affective lean toward intersubjectivity—to fill in the opening made through vulnerability.[37] It is moreover an invitation to take seriously the individuality of the illness-born humanism, this tiny needle that Franklin tries to thread against individualism and, now, against the person-less critique that leaves her undone in her encounter with debility. Individualism molded in the long and exploitative genealogy of liberalism and its postcolonial, imperial discontents offers no model for the ill; nor does the conservative humanism that requires its subjects to pretend laws, discourse, ideologies, and the toxic stream of "common sense" don't matter. But to do away with such toxic trapping by vacating the ill person the right to her complex personal testimony would result in the tragic triumph of structures of domination to make the already vulnerable subject to, rather than of, her relation to the regimes of (biomedical) power, of which her self story may be the only counternarrative available.

Malignant is a scholarly monograph, not a memoir by an academic. But as Jain acknowledges, it is the devastation of their personal encounter with cancer and biomedicine that deeply informs the work they perform in the book. They recall a point before the (mis)diagnosis of their own cancer meeting their partner's sister after her first chemotherapy session, during which they displayed their "unvarnished social aptitude with the ridiculous joke,

'Hey, you could totally be a lesbian!' I had picked up the culture of stigma, and this prevented me from genuinely recognizing her, even a few years later as she sat in a wheelchair shortly before her death."[38] Jain continues to offer a litany of ways that they, as a person yet untouched by cancer themself, were profoundly ill equipped to be in the presence of someone sick or dying as a member of that part of the social world that still held to the fantasy of indefinite health and restitution, as a citizen yet of the country, the "window into the larger social confusion about how illness fits in with the broader economic and political infrastructures that contour American ideas, even ideologies, of a lifespan."[39] Until they got sick, Jain was deeply invested in this imagination of this abstracted lifespan as their own, in which "the child survives the parent, the doctor survives the patient, the healthy survive the sick."[40] But illness and death and disability arrive at Franklin's threshold and put her argument into crisis; cells grow cancerous in Jain's body, and jokes about bald heads and queer passing become horrifically stale, because the suffering experienced is neither transferable nor transactional. It can only be experienced, and sometimes, if one pays enough attention, witnessed. *This* mode of experiencing and witnessing, both of which are singular acts (but that I contend can be—indeed, need to be—scalable), leads to an altogether different relation to what counts as analytically valuable, the individual and structural much more porous than we would normally allow or aver.

"People with cancer seemed like a different genre of person," writes Jain of themself, of course, antecedent to them being one of those people.[41] But once they become part of this genre, they take on new terms to forge their sense of personhood and sociality, and one might even go as far to say that they write the monograph with this newly hewn personhood in mind. In this different mode of writing, memoir joins with ethnography as Jain gathers with others who have experienced cancer to "'learn so much about' this or that. Yourself. What really matters. How much you love your family. How beautiful the little things are. . . . the recognition of grief and heartbreak."[42] All of them, by the way, very individual feelings for which an affect critic might scoff at such sentimentality of such an intimate public. But Jain pushes on insistently for this personhood that embraces what they feel and listens to what others feel: "And so we came together to discover community, to rediscover the selves that had been stolen by the cancer complex. A thirst emerged in the group, an unquenchable desire for new vocabulary, one that included suffering, but not victimhood; one that did not mimick [*sic*] conversations but rather reached for communication that mattered. We craved an alternative archive."[43] The metaphors of pedagogy and exploration that permeate Jain's prose to describe the desire that they and their companions with cancer undertake together in their shared spaces are reclamation projects, to wrest their narratives back from the bone-chilling cold of the clinic, but they are also vocabularies of critical affect that insist that the scholarly enterprise of criticism itself requires a way to do, say, materialism, but this time with feeling—a feeling, Jain would insist, that they can inhabit, and so can you.

Jain calls this an "elegiac politics—a stance that admits to the inevitability of [cancer deaths as a result of carcinogens] given the environmental and economic landscape [that] helps make this contradiction (okay, but not okay) not only legible, but livable and dieable. An elegiac politics demands the recognition of both enormous economic profits and enormous cultural and personal losses. An elegiac politics stares down the Game Face with the private face of cancer. Whether considered statistics or the victims of war, cancer's casualties are individual people."[44] Here, Jain speaks loudly where Franklin's voice falters in the wake of vulnerabilities born of illness, disability, and dying, which is the primacy of the individual as the *basis* for social diagnosis of what ails the institution itself: "I have aimed here to retrieve the individual—as a unit with specific features—from the aggregated thinking that contemporary cancer knowledge forces us into. . . . I want a new version of accounting, a bigger, richer vocabulary, and a voice to speak it with."[45] Rather than jettison the individual in the name of critique, as Franklin imagines is necessary but whose ghost in disabled form haunts her methodology, Jain asserts a claim for the individual suffering from cancer as the starting point for a methodology and, perhaps more important, a life practice allowing for a deeper disciplinary rigor that lets us see the built environment and witness the lives suffered within it, just as it gives space for building a social, political movement of people where singular stories are taken seriously, which are the only disciplines worth studying and movements worth following.

Mel Chen's New Materialisms and Political Ecology

Both illness and medicine are so all-consuming, so relentless in the flattening of the personhood on whom illness visits and medicine performs, that the labor of restoring to the self a story, a self-story, becomes a crucial dimension of taking account. To pay attention to the self is to exact a critical reading of the ecology of illness and the political economy of medicine, to see how the self is subjected to these two interrelated and imbricated regimes that cannot help but mandate living into a narrative not of the self's choosing, whether that of chaos's abyss or medicine's fantasies. Just as the physicians must rehabilitate themselves to regard their patients once again as fellow members of the same species; just as ill Asian Americans find themselves renarrating their value in the face of the body that fails them and thus compelling an inexorably different relation to the success frame of the model minority, so does the Asian American scholarly critic, professionally tasked with display-ing the erudition of critical exposure, recast what we had long jettisoned as old-fashioned and even reactionary: the recentering of the individual, not for the sake of liberal individualism, but to give the self a shape that can interact and be in relation with others—the agential vanguard of a transformative social imagination. Jain's insights and those of our other ill scholars rest on the restoration of the individual as the basis for such possibility.

Jain's personal experience with cancer leads them to move from regarding the ill as a "different genre of person" toward an affinity with illness's ontol-ogy, bearing the imprint of what they call an "elegiac politics"—that is, the contradiction of the "okay [and] not okay" of cancer "not only legible, but liv-able and dieable."[46] The elegiac in their politics makes for a reluctant, grimac-ing solidarity with their fellow wounded. Coeval with their cancer was an ill-ness suffered by Mel Chen, whose chronic condition not only circumscribed but also, tellingly, animated the argument of their first scholarly monograph, *Animacies: Biopolitics, Racial Mattering, and Queer Affect* (2012). The central concern of Chen's book, "How the fragile division between animate and in-animate—that is, beyond human and animal—is relentlessly produced and policed and maps important political consequences of that distinction," takes place first and foremost, as they narrate, in their own body.[47]

Late in the book, Chen reveals that their illness derives from the "effects of mercury toxicity," a condition that manifests in a variety of ways, including extreme sensitivity to other objects, seen and unseen, animate and inanimate. Chen's illness, they recall, can waylay them, leave them prone for countless hours and "anti-social" by socionormative expectations. But such sideways relations serve to underpin the entirety of their intellectual project, which is to consider how radical shifts in language's structure might impact how we structure the rest of the world—or, more polemically, to see how attention to representation can bear material effect, even politics. The first sentences of Chen's book express hope for as much, born from the intimacy of the body that they suffer: "Recently, after reaching a threshold of 'recovery' from a chronic illness—an illness that has affected me not only physically, but spatially, familially, economically, and socially, and set me on a long road of thinking about the marriage of bodies and chemicals—I found myself deeply suspicious of my own reassuring statements to my anxious friends that I was feeling more alive again."[48] Chen's suspicion toward their own language, ut-terances designed to assuage "anxious friends" that they were getting better, in effect to restore to them statements that affirm the fiction of restitution, hints at their incredulity to such reassurance, given how much their impact affects people and environs beyond just their own body, a "recovery" that is also a "long road."

But perhaps more important for Chen's intellectual and political investments, such "statements"—which, after all, are ways of structuring the world through language, which itself is their primary mode of scholarly engagement, trained as they were in linguistics at Berkeley—Chen's suspicion remains even if they were indeed feeling "more alive again" in their "recovery":

> Surely I had been no *less* alive when I was *more* sick, except under the accountings of an intuitive and immediately problematic notion of "liveliness" and other kinds of "freedom" and "agency." I felt unsettled not only for reasons of disability politics—for "lifely wellness" colludes with a logic that troublingly naturalizes illness's morbidity—but also because I realized that in the most containing and altered moments of illness, as often occurs with those who are severely ill, I came to know an incredible wakefulness, one that I was now paradoxically losing and could only try to commit to memory.[49]

Here Chen affirms one of the key insights of disability studies: that able-bodiedness is correlated to liveliness only by means of the socially normative enforcement of a hierarchy of value based on the purported productivity and activity of some bodies over others, Parsons's "sick role" the temporary exception from such productivity with the promise of future activity. A chronically ill or disabled person, however, she sees herself or is seen along this spectrum—is viewed, by default—as deformed from the able-bodied norm. Chen, however, asserts further that it is only *through* their illness that they achieved heightened consciousness, the "incredible wakefulness" that gave them insight that was not possible before or after. The chaos of illness begets illumination.

This insight structures not just Chen's argument but, more ambitiously, their utopian political hope, which is enabled by the very matters (or toxins, as they will reveal later) that engendered their illness in the first place. The ostensibly inanimate objects that circulate in Chen's body are the conditions for their heightened liveliness or animacy. This mutual symbiosis is the basis for a thorough revisitation of the very nature of ontological order:

> Using animacy . . . helps us theorize current anxieties around the production of humanness in contemporary times, particularly with regard to humanity's partners in definitional crime: animality (as its

analogue or limit), nationality, race, security, environment, and sexuality. Animacy activates new theoretical formations that trouble and undo stubborn binary systems of difference, including dynamism/stasis, life/death, subject/object, speech/nonspeech, human/animal, natural body/cyborg. In its more sensitive figurations, animacy has the capacity to rewrite conditions of intimacy, engendering different communalisms and revising biopolitical spheres, or, at least, how we might theorize them.[50]

We can pause for a moment at Chen's final qualifier: that the radical potential for imagining the world through the lens of animacy rather than binarisms built on ableist anthropocentrisms may remain more theoretical than material. We can pause, but we can also follow where they want us to go with them, what Chen hopes for through their scholarly project: which is to foreground their ill body as an example of how a wounded, vulnerable, and deeply imbricated body can be a sign of an altogether different rubric for sociality as such.

But to get to their ill body requires a journey through what Chen calls the normative animacy hierarchy as established by anthropocentrism, beginning with the modes of human interaction through the human and nonhuman animal threshold, and concluding with those things in the world viewed as inanimate: metals. Chen's chapters move first through the "political grammar" of the animacy hierarchy by exposing how language works to reinforce relations of power, even when discussing insurgent possibilities such as the contemporary *reanimation* of the term "queer." From this consideration of how and what humans call one another, Chen pivots to the nexus of human and animal, which, they argue, is deeply invested in questions of race and nation, whether highlighting the animalizing of the Chinese immigrant in the nineteenth century in securing U.S. white American humanity or demonstrating how theorizing sexuality and animality gesture to how "animacy *itself* can be queer, for animacy can work to blur the tenuous hierarchy of human-animal-vegetable-mineral with which it is associated."[51] Finally, Chen moves to lead and the racial politics that inhere in the moral panic in 2007 over toys manufactured in China that were suffused with lead and the greater fear that children putting those objects in their mouths might simultaneously be poisoned and (racially) marked by them as much as they might (queerly) enjoy this action. All this is to say that, to get to Chen (especially for a "first book," which Chen's was), we needed to move through the classic ephemera of academic scholarship. Language, historical archive, and popular media all serve as Chen's unsurprising cultural studies bailiwick. This is meant not to minimize this important, trenchant work, but simply to acknowledge the necessity of signposting the scholarly genre's citational expectations.

And then Chen's sixth chapter, "Following Mercurial Affect," arrives, beginning with the ominous truism, "Toxins are everywhere."[52] For the next two thousand words or so, Chen rehearses what reads as conventional accounts of toxicity, in both their physical manifestation and effect and their metaphorical usage and the affects of toxicity. Thus, for example, "All cultural productions of toxicity must be rethought as an integral part of the affective fabric of immunity nationalism."[53] As in previous chapters, Chen lays bare how animacy hierarchies work to make (inorganic) toxins the "biopolitical entrainment as an instrument of difference" as they wend their way through (organic) bodies.[54] They then offer a queer, provisional reversal of the subject-object relations born of toxicity: like Anatole Broyard's intoxication by his illness, Chen hints at intoxification as a blurring of the immunity-toxicity divide, which then leads to this luminous argument in the form of assertion: "It seems never a simple matter to discuss toxicity, to objectify it. It is yet another matter to experience something that seems by one measure or another to be categorized as a toxin, to undergo intoxication, intoxification. This difference raises questions about toxic methodology, which in some way inherits anthropology's question about what to do to respond to crises of objectivity."[55] Chen is, of course, referring to questions popularized some decades ago by men such as Clifford Geertz and Johannes Fabian, but whose revolution was begun by anthropologists in feminist, Third World, and subaltern studies who questioned the epistemological foundations of a field devoted to "knowing" human worlds. To develop a method of understanding toxicity *as a toxic subject themself*, Chen suggests, is to slough off the pretense that haunts even the most radical cultural studies projects—or, as Chen asks, "How can we think more broadly about synthesis and symbiosis, including toxic vapors, interspersals, intrinsic mixings, and alterations, favoring interabsorption over corporeal exceptionalism? I will not address these questions from the point of view of mythic health."[56] If the animacy hierarchy, at bottom, serves a logic of binarism that, as Jacques Derrida taught us back in his heyday, underpins Western thought—subject and object as basic syntax—then Chen cannot continue to make a utopian argument without a methodology that gets at this binarism as *the* problem of knowledge and of action itself. A methodological approach to toxicity, a toxic methodology to the ordering of the world, demands the undoing of this order. Chen must make themself the "tale" from which critical knowledge derives. They are simultaneously the *subject* of knowledge and the *knowing* subject: Chen embodies toxic methodology, and this, they suggest, is the method of knowing par excellence.

"I theorize toxicity as it has profoundly impacted my own health, my queerness," Chen writes to begin their tale. A startling statement about archive, method, and ethics: their body is the text through which their theory of toxicity develops; generalized, any theorization of toxicity with fidelity must begin there. Chen does so not without trepidation, as they lay out before making this statement of theorization that stems from their ill subjectivity: "I move now from a theoretical discussion of metaphors about threat into what feels, for me personally, like riskier terrain, the terrain of the autobiographical. As academics are often trained to avoid writing in anything resembling a confessional mode, such a turn is fraught with ambivalence."[57] Chen does not dwell on their ambivalence or their feeling of risk. Suffice it to say, however, that they shed a significant light on the work of academic criticism as a genre of risk taking, except that it is generally not the critic who bears the weight of the risk; thus the critic often doesn't feel the freight and fraughtness of ambivalence. That risk is generally borne by the object of the critic's gaze, which begs the questions: What does it mean for the academic enterprise *not* to put oneself as the academic at risk of analysis *before* subjecting anyone else through such mediation? What remains laconic in the ethics of academic training that one's own story of vulnerable embodiment feels dangerous in a way that doesn't when we turn our critical sights onto others and expect them to do the critical dirty work for us? Chen exposes the ethics of textual risk taking by telling the story of their illness and insisting, lightly but insistently, that a methodology worth its ethical salt must start from there. Chen calls this invocation of their ill autobiography a "complementary kind of knowledge production" to those they examined in previous chapters, but it is this personal experience with illness that produces something far more transformative than any work of cultural studies scholarship could have provided: "My repository of thoughts, experiences, and theorizations while ill—*ones that queerly and profoundly changed my relationship to intimacy*—could be considered a kind of 'archive of feelings,' to use Ann Cvetkovich's important terminology."[58] Intimacy in all of its permutations—sexuality, desire, embodiment, affect, an identity among them—comes to the fore in the crucible of ill experience, a profane illumination of the very nature of sociality and social ordering, as changing one's notion of intimacy has implications for the question of relationality as such.

The toxicity that inhabits Chen's body is not voluntary but the result of years of exposure to mercury; it is also neither solely negative nor pleasurable in "recognizable terms." Rather, their disposition to the world remains radically and mutably altered. Describing a day of relative "well being," Chen recounts the heightened awareness they must navigate in public, including, but not exhausted by, the odors of cologne or cigarette smoke; intrusive stares or comments by strangers (To what? Their face mask? Their race? Their gender presentation? Chen can't tell; taunts from their childhood overdetermine their interpretation of the present moment); whether or not to name and share their condition with others or whether or not to try to "pass" as normatively able at the moment, however precarious the moment is. The struggle to keep track of what to keep track of is exhausting and potentially debilitating, and it is for this reason—at the least and notwithstanding the physiological effects of their body's toxicity—that Chen arrives at a wholly different notion of embodiment, in which fluidity and uncertainty are better descriptive terms than anything resembling settled identity: "Given my condition, I must constantly renegotiate, and recalibrate, my embodied experiences of intimacy, altered affect, and the porousness of the body."[59] It is the latter experience of porousness that determines Chen's changed relation to intimacy and affect, as their body simply cannot absorb new, everyday toxins, consumed as their body is by extant mercury. They are as a result affectively "mercurial," given to what they call "unstable and wildly unpredictable" behavior—or, at least, what we might consider as such from the vantage of normative human sociability. Chen's toxicity makes them recoil from their lover's touch, which they remember with a certain horror for having been a "bad" partner, but this scene highlights a crucial reorientation to their social geography. "Humans are to a radical degree no longer the primary cursors of my physical inhabitation of space," Chen writes. "Inanimate things take on a greater, holistic importance. It also means that I am perpetually itinerant, even when I have a goal; it means I will never walk in a straight line. There are also lessons here, reminders of interdependency, of softness, of fluidity, of receptivity, of immunity's fictivity and attachment's impermanence; life sustains even—or especially—in this kind of silence, this kind of pause, this dis-ability."[60] This provisional reversal of the animacy hierarchy—their preference for the haptic embrace of the inanimate couch over their human lover's—seems "unbelievable" in the aftermath of Chen's illness, after they have recovered to a state approximating "health."

But the existential and visceral states of health and illness cannot fully demarcate what Chen discovered during their most toxic moments: that the objects along the animacy spectrum, whether couch, plant, cat, stranger, friend, or lover, are "all the same ontological thing." Chen writes, "But it is only in the recovering of my human-directed sociality that the couch really becomes an unacceptable partner. This episode, which occurs again and again, forces me to rethink animacy, since I have encountered an intimacy that does not differentiate, is not dependent on a heartbeat. The couch and I are interabsorbent, interporous, and not only because the couch is made of mammalian skin."⁶¹ Chen's highlighting of the state of recovery as a return to a form of sociality that privileges the human echoes the arguments put forth by critical ethnic, gender, and disability studies, all of which provide exposures to the hierarchies embedded in which forms of sociality are privileged in social worlds created by the logics of racism, sexism, and ableism. Conversely, to fantasize a world in which the couch *is* an acceptable partner for Chen gestures especially to the insight of disability studies as to how a more expansive understanding of what constitutes the "good" body can provide new possibilities of "good" modes of relationality beyond fetishisms of autonomy and heroic independence.⁶² Chen's recurring experiences of interobject relation, born of their toxic animation, thus forms the central kernel of their argument, which begins with their preoccupation with language but moves toward what they call worlding—that is, how they describe this world and how they might live in it: "If language normally and habitually distinguishes human and inhuman, live and dead, but then in certain circumstances wholly fails to do so, what might this tell us about the porosity of biopolitical logics themselves?"⁶³ What, indeed, might Chen's toxic body tell about porosity and possibility that a "healthy" one, even one as academically trained as theirs, never can? Chen is asking us to imagine an otherwise not possible if we dwell in world of strict human valuation and, by extension, a valuation of humanity itself based on how "well" or nontoxic a life we are living.

To this, Chen lets fly their theoretical and political imagination: "In perhaps its best versions, toxicity does not repel but propels queer loves, especially once we release it from exclusively human hosts, disproportionately inviting dis/ability, industrial labor, biological targets, and military vaccine recipients [all figures of negative animacy in previous chapters]—inviting loss and its 'losers' and trespassing containers of animacy."⁶⁴ In invoking "loss and its 'losers,'" Chen gestures to Jack Halberstam's "queer art of failure," a theoretical suspicion of resistance's triumph that merely reinscribes formations of power around other celebrated subjects rather than rejects the very logic of success even in the name of a movement, community, or identity.⁶⁵ This "best version" of toxicity's potential certainly requires disability studies' insistence on shattering any normative figurations of human experience or embodiment, as well as tender attention to experiences of vulnerability born of normativity's oppression. The "queer love" for humanity's and animacy's losers alike that comes from Chen's symbiotic, if vexed, relation to the toxicities that *both* pain them and make them miserable at times *and* invite them to see the world in wholly new and transformed ways opens us to imagine and perhaps embody, even practice, social relations that cannot possibly be managed or maintained by biomedicine's binarisms and specializations. To this, Chen acknowledges the charge that this rearticulated theory of the body, of ethics and desire, of politics and worlding, seems hopelessly, even ridiculously, utopian, especially given their testimony about how exhausting and painful their toxic condition can be. Chen's illness is a locus of suffering as much as it is a window to a new world. Indeed, they insist that their affection for toxicity cannot stand in for utopia, given its "screamingly negative affects," a description that reads for me as intimately and intensely autobiographical.

Still, why not follow along with Chen's logic to its utopian end, insofar as theory always has embedded within it such impulses for such idealized telos, poststructuralist inoculatory skepticism notwithstanding? Chen's experience with toxicity is uncommon but not rare, and certainly their generalized condition of chronic illness, pain, and environmental sensitivities shares cognates with those who suffer other illnesses. Why not find a way to idealize these conditions, to find the art, if you will, in pathology? Chen's toxicity aligns them with other forms of social vulnerability produced by forces that demand hierarchy—race, gender, sexuality, ableism among them, for sure. In *this* sense, "in assuming both individual and collective vulnerability, it suggests an ulterior ethical stance."[66] Such a differential ethics of relating to objects in a leaky, porous way, and thereby inviting a sociality with other humans in analogously leaky, porous ways, invites us also to imagine a wholly differential politics in which to materialize this utopian impulse. Take Chen's operative term of coexistence with a nonhuman object, toxicity, and replace it with other terms mobilized in medicine as its enemy—disease, cancer, infection, morbidity, and keep going—and then substitute them in this sentence: "If we were to release toxicity from its own stalwart anti-ness, its ready definition as an unwelcome guest, it has the possibility to intervene into the binary between the segregated fields of 'life' and 'death,' vitality and morbidity."[67] Now think how Chen's embodied theory would make practically every metaphor medicine demands we use to describe illness—whether it's a war on cancer or battling an infection or turning a patient into a fighter—inherently violent and *unethical.* To imagine illness or disease not as a condition in which eradication is the desired goal but, instead, as a form of coexistence is either horrifying or utopian. Chen asks us to theorize and then imagine living into the latter.

In their concluding reflections, Chen remembers a prompt from Jacqui Alexander, who asks a question regarding the ethics and politics of the academic enterprise in regard to its relation to the *longue durée* of the animacy hierarchy, which is also a history of "the seat and time of empire": "What can we do as intellectuals within and without academies from the seat of empire, particularly to encounter the problem of the 'here and now' versus the 'then and there' that colonial and imperial time naturalize?"[68] Chen names their academic vocation "eclectic," citing their "feral" transdisciplinary and their affinity with queer of color and disability/crip intellectual and political communities. I suggest that central to Chen's eclecticism is their assertion that their own body theorizes and manifests the problem of the here and now versus then and there by doing as much as possible to shorten the distance between the critic and their object, the critic as their object, deserving of queer love and care, as much love and care as Chen had for their couch. It is a paradoxical commitment to the animacy even of death-dealing illness that, finally, "encourages opening to the senses of the world, receptivity, vulnerability."[69] Chen wonders whether their readers might want to live there. I wonder what the consequences are if we don't want to.

Cancer, Reparations, and the Bardo of Dying: Lana Lin

Chen's call for communing with all things without prejudice, to contemplate attachment and vulnerability to the inanimate as a radical form of queer love, to be in love even with those elements toxic to their very body, are not only cited but held up as a methodological ideal in Lana Lin's monograph *Freud's Jaw and Other Lost Objects: Fractured Subjectivity in the Face of Cancer* (2017). Lin's psychoanalytic study of three public intellectuals—Sigmund Freud, Audre Lorde, and Eve Kosofsky Sedgwick—not only aligns with Chen's critique of the animacy hierarchy and binarism of life and death but also, significantly, finds inspiration in Chen's insertion of their personal story as central to their method and theory. Calling Chen's example the "autopathographic impulse," Lin writes, "I punctuate *Freud's Jaw* with observations collected from my experience with breast cancer."[70] Like Chen's, Lin's experience of illness is her opening to vulnerability and the starting point of her theoretical reflection; unlike Chen, though, who barely makes mention of their interface with medicine, Lin, because of her cancer, has to wrestle with the agents of medicine, who, like our medical writers and those who give care to our ill authors, continue to insist on being the primary definers and monopolizers of the language of illness, Lin's included. Her experience with breast cancer is made conscious and given its name at the doctor's office. "Upon diagnosis," Lin recounts, "I initially underwent a nipple-sparing mastectomy, whose name, although not commonly known, ought to be self-explanatory. When the pathology report indicated that the margins were not clear, that is, that the knife that presumably drew a line between cancer and not-cancer came too close to the cancerous side for everyone to feel comfortable, I was ultimately advised to have what is called a 'completion mastectomy.'"[71] Note here the manner in which Lan casts herself as the patient, devoid of action, rendered to the passive voice while the medical texts—the definitive name of the procedure, the action and authority of the pathology report, the finality of medical advice—take up her world and culminate in what she will focus on: the term "completion mastectomy," which will serve as the medicalized anchor from which her argument contrapuntally moves forward, as a polemic against the very idea of completion.

Lin notes that only someone so steeped in medical discourse as her surgeon wouldn't see the absurd irony of calling a procedure "completion mastectomy," as if "one would become more complete as a consequence of the further removal of parts of oneself."[72] But the paradox of affect here, the finality of a medical goal juxtaposed with the resigned horror of this goal's material effect, which is the further amputation of one's body as a sign of completion, conjures for Lin a question that wonders about the "very idea of what constitutes completion": "Completion may consist of the feeling— whether it is illusory or fantasy—of wholeness, a kind of psychic completion wherein the body and psyche are for the most part aligned."[73] Here Lin calls the feeling of embodied completion—what Frank calls the restitution narrative, based on either illusion or fantasy—a being duped by a false narrative or living into a self-consciously fictitious one. Both the medical promise that a procedure will bring one back to a state of indefinite health and the narrative medicine demands that completion as bodily health is not only normal but the only socially acceptable condition are called into question as ontological and, perhaps, ethical conditions. Cancer irrevocably shatters this illusion/ fantasy for Lin, and illness more generally presents a more foundational precondition to the basic tenets of human life, not as moving toward completion but as a movement that is perpetually partial.

Thus, Lin invests in psychoanalysis, whose epistemology expunges anything that approximates what she calls completion or what we might call wholeness or arrival. Consider Lin's argument for the book, and bear in mind her brief telling of her cancer diagnosis and treatment:

> I consider the ways in which cancer exposes a person to the vulner-
> ability of her perceived bodily integrity and agency, rupturing her
> sense of wholeness as a human being with a degree of control over
> her body parts and the presumed continuities of life. Cancer not only
> complicates the ideal of wholeness in which people are physically
> and psychically invested, but it also unveils the unwanted knowledge
> that from the outset we have never been entirely whole, a knowledge

that most of us repress in order to function from day to day. In short, cancer shows the hole in the whole.[74]

Like Chen's toxic body, Lin's cancerous body manifests a profane illumination of a knowledge that needs to be repressed for society to function: the lie of completion and the lie of indefinite health. In short, the "hole in the whole" is the kernel of death and mortality in the fictive narrative of immortality that we want to continue to tell and that medicine promises us with its fingers crossed. The fundamental rupture at the heart of human psyche and a person's very sense of subjectivity, which underpins the heart of psychoanalysis, is for Lin the vocation of cancer, the illness and existential condition that ruptures wholeness as illusory or fantasy. This realization of cancer's and psychoanalysis's proximity to partiality and vulnerability forms Lin's argument, for sure, but it also catalyzes the very act of writing. She documents this in the first paragraph of her acknowledgments section, which also serves as a kind of afterword: "This book evolved, quite frankly, out of a breast cancer diagnosis that came during my second year of pursuing my doctorate. It was a life-altering event that followed a different set of life-altering events. . . . In the meantime, I continued to make films and art, and I trained as a psychoanalyst for three years."[75] Both the creative dimensions of art and the resistance to consolidation in psychoanalysis give Lin a venue through which to find a "coherence of fragmentary pieces of our lives and worlds," which is different from completion. The book that she creates and that her readers hold in their hands is "probably a culmination of speaking out my fears and desires, of transforming silence into a language that loosely holds [her] together."[76]

It is the "loosely" constituted dimension of psychoanalytic language that Lin is drawn to, insofar as the genealogy of its theory and practice give her a language to make sense of something as life-altering as cancer that can attend to the illness's shattering effects. Psychoanalysis, after all, assumes neither affective stasis nor mental satisfaction. Instead, like the anxieties born of illness, it "conceptualizes not only metastatic disease [whether neurosis or cancer], but also the idea of recurrence, the absence of cure, the presence of death or proximity to one's mortality."[77] This may suggest that Lin is drawn principally to negative affect, but her aim, crucially, is akin to that of others who live with cancer, whether in full-blown metastatic disease or its remission: to find a way to craft a reparative narrative if restitution is no longer or really never was available. Lin hopes to recuperate the "melancholia" of psychanalysis's emphasis on the centrality of loss "for a politics of creativity": "Only by attending to, rather than disavowing, perennial loss can we as a culture and as a collection of lost objects ourselves, refind ourselves, love one another, and labor toward physical, emotional, and political reparations."[78] Insofar as the "best" one can hope for in a psychoanalytic framework is not the eradication of symptoms derived from neurotic subjectivity but the process to develop a symptom that one can "enjoy" rather than suffer, Lin regards the theoretical disposition of psychoanalysis as deeply analogous to living with an illness such as cancer: illness is a kind of neurotic structure from which there is no escape, so how might one "enjoy" one's illness, a sentiment that Broyard expresses as a form of intoxication? To "refind," love, and labor toward reparations requires a kind of labor akin to the therapeutic work that psychoanalysis demands of its practitioners, an attention to the "holes" in one's psyche out of which a better symptomatology emerges. Psychoanalysis and illness both invite those who inhabit their respective worlds to new forms of enjoyment.

But we need to be even more specific, because Lin insists that it is the specific form of illness that is cancer that haunts psychoanalysis. Cancer structures this field; it is perhaps the primal symptom of psychoanalysis: "Cancer has a psychoanalytic meaning. Cancer has a meaning for the body of psychoanalysis. It bears repeating that it is not any disease that has cast its shadow upon psychoanalytic history and theory. It is specifically cancer that plagues psychoanalysis as 'unwelcome intruder.'"[79] So Lin undertakes throughout her monograph an episodic genealogy of this relation between a disease and a theory of mind and practice of life by highlighting the work of three thinkers and writers who develop through their cancer experiences a "subjectivity of survival," which she views as the goal of psychoanalysis, to survive in the face of profound loss. In considering the first of these, Lin develops the notion of "not death," a reading of Freud's death drive as a "paradoxical entanglement of the life and death drives and a mode of survival," which in turn forms the foundational language of Freudian psychoanalytic theory.[80] Freud's life with mouth cancer and the prostheses that he would have to wear from 1924 until his death in 1939 became somatic reminders of his own mortality, an embodied paradoxical entanglement of his life attached to emblems of his finitude, the cancer and the nonhuman object supplementing the part of him that was removed because of the disease. "Physical decomposition dispossesses the psyche," writes Lin. Bodily decay makes one a stranger to one's sense of self as a reflex of disavowal: this can't be me, and yet it is. Freud calls this strangeness *unheimlich*, which we translate as *uncanny*. It is from and through cancer, Lin argues, that Freud envisioned the very structure of the psyche in psychoanalysis: "Cancerous deterioration unhouses Freud and turns his bodily inhabitance into a disruptive intermingling of living and dying. Freud names this process as uncanny, the uncanniness of being both oneself and not oneself. . . . Cancer's special uncanniness brings to light what ought to be hidden, and it continually recurs or threatens to return."[81] Cancer, as illness, interrupts how one tells the story of one's body, demands a new narrative in the aftermath of the wreckage, and erupts and disrupts the sheen of psychic health. It reveals the wreckage that are the elements of the psychic structure, the "not-me" at the center of the self.

Lin continues to elaborate and connect what she calls, borrowing from Derrida, the "autothanatography of psychoanalysis," psychoanalysis as kind of biography of cancer, which is "not only due to its founder's protracted malady": "Cancer reflects the paradoxical double meanings of the not-death drive. It names a persistent dread, anxiety, and fear of inner disintegration that is encountered by many psychoanalysts and may be innate to human beings. It is also identified with unceasing proliferation, *jouissance*, and the drive toward immortality."[82] Freud's cancer gives him insight into the antagonisms at the heart of psychic, even biological, human life: Eros and Thanos, love/life and death as primal drives whose oscillation forms the antagonism and antinomies of life itself. Cancer is killing me, but I want to live forever; the part of me that can live forever is cancer, which is the part that will kill me.

There is for Lin a more intimate connection to Freud's cancer and, more specifically, to his ambivalent attachment to his prosthetic devices, which is presented as her analogous struggle over whether she should submit to breast reconstruction following her mastectomy. She relates that, when declining reconstructive surgery because of her unease about having a foreign object in her body, her (male) surgeon "replied, nonplussed, 'You have fillings, don't you?'" The take-for-granted seamlessness of coexistence between organic and inorganic matter in one's body that characterizes Lin's surgeon's view of breast reconstruction cannot account for the general condition of unease, her sense of the bodily uncanniness, that makes this kind of coexistence fraught. Lin may indeed have fillings, but the question of reconstructive surgery of her breasts, the site of trauma and the general unsettling of her psyche thanks to cancer, is hardly a reproducible daily event: "the struggle that ensues can be felt as a process of technological dehumanization."[83] So whereas for Freud the prosthetic object serves as a stand-in for the "not death" of psychoanalysis-*cum*-cancer, for Lin the threat of the prosthetic breast becomes a sign of being relegated to the nonhuman, a sentiment that aligns her with Lorde's own struggles with breast cancer *and* the imperative toward prosthetic reconstruction. Indeed, while Lin's chapter on Lorde ostensibly focuses on a Kleinian reading of the writer-activist's oeuvre, she highlights the shared struggle of having to fight the medical and broader cultural injunction to consent to reconstructive surgery, which Lorde describes in *Cancer Journals* as a "prosthetic pretense" to normative expectations to which she refused to submit. For Lorde, Lin suggests (and as we saw in the previous chapter), a breast prosthesis serves as little more than a "false advertisement that the body in question had not undergone any change and that the postmastectomy woman should still be regarded as the same woman she had been prior to surgery" because of the cosmetic pretense of normatively symmetrically shaped breasts.[84] Lin even recounts that this same breast surgeon relates an anecdote that he'd forgotten he had performed reconstructive surgery on a woman and wondered, upon learning of her recent delivery of a baby, whether she was breastfeeding.

Lin regards her surgeon's story as an example of Kleinian fetish, "an overvalued, trauma-induced object that conceals an underlying gender confusion."[85] But it is in this rehearsal of her surgeon's story of another woman that we see her align herself with Lorde's critique of the social dimensions of the fetishism of breast reconstruction. The "gender confusion" that the reconstructed breast tries to mask is the one that insists on a sliver of a figuration of femininity that is assumed cis and hetero and maybe even coded white. The shocked woman's response, "Why, of course not, doctor!" highlights the imagined idealization of this woman as having secured what Lee Edelman would call the reproductive futurity of cis-hetero (white) womanhood that the surgeon wants to maintain, if not at all costs, then at least with considerable determination. In one of Lorde's *Cancer Journals* axioms, "We were never meant to survive," we might read Lin's deep identification with Lorde's disidentification with this idealization. Given that the elevation of the woman submitting to breast reconstruction—in Lorde's day, and even when Lin was faced with the same choice/demand—implicitly and oftentimes explicitly, as Lorde recounts of her experiences, diminishes the value and experiences of those who cannot or will not conform to these expectations, Lin finds in a fellow queer woman of color a related feeling of being made object, inanimate, de-human: "The 'no-breasted' postmastectomy woman, the person of color, the gender nonconforming, the disabled, the poor, and the old, each of these subjects are ejected as foreign objects from a society that can only perceive of difference as endangering."[86] If cancer and the prosthetic objects that remind one of his disease are for Freud (and Lin) material emblems of the antagonisms and ambivalences of the psyche in psychoanalysis, then cancer and the imperative for the prosthetic breast are for Lorde (and Lin) part of a semiotic that register raced, gendered, and other embodied elements from which they are categorically expunged as less valued or unvalued by medicine. It is not only that Lorde and Lin are different; it is their insistence on their difference, their refusal of medicine's "corrective," that make them in the eyes of biomedicine both endangering and revolting.

In the face of such loathing over their difference and their refusal of gender conformity, however, a "house of difference" is possible. Lorde makes her "different kind of body" an object to be fetishized by others, which, Lin argues, is her ultimate contribution, even sacrifice. "Lorde offers herself to her black sisters," Lin continues, "as she would medicine to the ill or a tool for useful production."[87] In her refusal to adopt the reconstructed breast as a fetish that tries to undo the gender uncertainty of the postmastectomy woman, Lorde transforms her body-in-difference into its own fetish, and Lin agrees that Lorde "is used fetishistically by queers of color today . . . the lesbian/poet/mother warrior encourages her community to use her as a tool, as a fetish."[88] It is Lorde's "self-love" of her postmastectomy body, a body rendered differentially as Black, queer, and ill, that then becomes the condition for a "strange space of difference, modeling how mothers might cannily reclaim themselves as the uncanny original site of home."[89] In psychoanalytic terms, Lorde becomes her own better symptom.[90] This creative impulse that stems from the destructive impulses of both cancer and the social response to fetishize the loss the illness engenders moves Lin to make use of flights of imagination to create for herself an idea, an object, however fanciful, to engage meaningfully the crisis wrought by cancer. Prior to her diagnosis, she relates dreaming of her body gaining a new organ, which she calls a "keen," and speculates whether it serves as an "anticipatory recompense for the loss [she would] suffer" in the wake of diagnosis. She discovers later the term's connection to death and grief and realizes that the dream of her keen aligns with what she views as Lorde's writerly vocation through her illness, which is to "think creatively and critically about the meaning of bodily absence, corporeal suffering, and defamiliarization . . . , putting death to use such that survival amounts to an insistence upon 'not-death.'"[91] From the "not death" of Freud, Lin learns the nether region that the psyche inhabits between the dueling drives of Eros and Thanos; Lorde's "not death" teaches Lin to insist on living—through the creative act—even though, as a fellow queer woman of color, a queer Asian American woman, she, too, is not really meant to survive. Lin's "keen" is both a creative act and an emblem against which she survives, the primal organ of loss and finitude: "I give myself language in naming an imaginary part of myself 'keen.' My keen, like Lorde's and [Adrienne] Rich's poetry, might be regarded as a creation that can be used for mourning absence, that symbolizes but does not substitute for the lost object."[92]

There's more here than Lorde authorizing Lin's agency to give herself a fictive organ and an imaginary language to create an object that attends to her mourning of her body altered by cancer. For even as she meditates on Lorde's work via Kleinian psychoanalysis, Lin acknowledges that she must undertake this reading against the grain, given that Melanie Klein could not imagine a psychoanalytic theory with a queer Black woman in mind. Lorde is beyond the sociological imagination of Klein's psychoanalytic method.[93] In bringing them together, then, Lin wishes not only to reveal elements of the two that are unavailable when one highlights their "incompatibilities," but also, more important, to assert that Lorde's subjectivity, not imagined by those who created the infrastructural textbook, deserves the depth and complexity of human psychology. In insisting on an interior life that mirrored Lorde's social struggles as a queer Black woman, Lin drags psychoanalysis away from the cis, white, and heteronormative figures that underpin its genealogy toward those to whom she is politically and affectively committed, those who also deserve a deep psychic life that matches the complexity of their sociology. One might go as far as to say that Lorde overshadows the patriarchs and matriarchs of psychoanalysis, which, in turn, enables Lin to imagine psychoanalysis as a proximate language for her cancer and her cancer as the experience through which psychoanalytic realism takes on credence. Chronicling a moment during the writing of *Freud's Jaw*, during which her dentist discovers a lesion on her tongue, she wonders first about overidentifying with Freud and the lesions that marked his cancer of the mouth. But she then speculates on a series of *disidentifications*—with Freud, psychoanalysis, even her cancer now in remission—because of the seeming incompatibility of *her* identity with psychoanalysis's historical interlocutors: "Freud's name is often associated with a conservatism that goes against the grain of my interests as a queer woman of color. Diagnosed with cancer at the same age that Audre Lorde was when her malignant tumor was discovered, and like her having had my right breast removed, at times I have felt, as she did, that I was never meant to survive. But I am reminded that Lorde addresses the problem of survival in the plural, intoning that *we* were never meant to survive."[94] Here, Lin invokes José Esteban Muñoz's theory of disidentification as a queer strategy for survival and suggests that Lorde does so similarly for Lin's investment's in psychoanalysis: if "disidentification is about managing and negotiating historical trauma and systemic violence," which include the traumas and violence of the very psychoanalytic method to which she is committed, Lin advances Lorde's insistence on surviving despite expectation as a way, following Muñoz, to "tactically and simultaneously work on, with, and against, a cultural form [such as psychoanalysis]."[95] Caring for those never meant to survive, and mourning either those who didn't survive or for survivors mourning what is lost in such survival becomes both a "creative form of care" and a "labor of care," whose "black heart [following Lorde and Saidiya Hartman] . . . pulses in the bardo of dying, making possible the prospect of productive relation."⁹⁶ Lorde's "black heart" gives Lin's Asian American story of cancer a pedagogical and political purpose.

This "bardo of dying" that Lin references comes from her consideration of Sedgwick's long deliberation with cancer, which manifested in various modes of writing, including the memoiristic, the scholarly-critical, and even forms that approach the religious and spiritual. Originating in the Tibetan Buddhist tradition, the bardo constitutes a state of existence—like "dying, meditation, sleep, and dreams"—between consciousness and nonexistence, a gap, if you will, "in which the possibility of realization is heightened."⁹⁷ This religiously inflected emblem, this liminal state aligned with dying as a stage between life and death, becomes Sedgwick's domain, one that she cannily and deliberately develops as a mode of scholarship that requires attention to knowledge that is possible *only* through illness—specifically, incurable, terminal illness. To witness someone dying is to learn something wholly new, to be taught something that can't be taught anywhere else. Such witness is a form of pedagogy that, for Lin, makes Sedgwick a central figure in the work of letting illness guide the scholarly endeavor. Lin cites no less than Lauran Berlant, whose deep critique of "intimate publics" might cast Sedgwick's performance with more than a bit of critical regard, skeptical as she is of rhetoric and affects of intimacy. But, as a reminder that we were here before, way back in the Introduction, Berlant says this about Sedgwick's memoir, which includes her cancer struggle and the conversations with her therapist surrounding her illness: "Eve's work is a training in being in the room with that ambivalence, which she also called unbearable, in its revelation that having and losing are indistinguishable."⁹⁸ Berlant's "a training" is, for Lin, a statement of Sedgwick's writing about illness as a form of pedagogy. "Sedgwick points out," Lin goes on to write, "that the insights that illness can give on the processes of living and dying have long functioned as master teachings: 'the sickbed or deathbed is continually produced as a privileged scene of teaching.' What she calls the 'pedagogy of illness and dying' can short circuit temporal expectations of vitality and destabilize customary relations between teachers and students. For instance, the young student dying of AIDS can advise the older professor who has been diagnosed with cancer."⁹⁹ To write through the liminality of cancer becomes the contemporary privileged scene of teaching, the scholarly account of terminal illness the academic's version of the deathbed, which demands of its readers who wish to remain in the room critical silence, the discourse of critique hushed to let the dying reveal her insights without interruption.

To bring one as trenchant as Berlant to a kind of awed pause is what Sedgwick infers as "reparative reading," which I touched on in Chapter 2.

To rehearse and extend the idea: this mode of reading is less a method than an observational disposition that Sedgwick takes up toward the end of her *Touching Feeling: Affect, Pedagogy, Performativity* (2003). It is reparation that is central to Lin's monograph, a form not only of thinking, reading, and writing, but of living as a kind of afterlife to the loss of restoration, of the body after cancer and of the psyche after the losses cancer produces. In her chapter on reparative reading, Sedgwick provides the example of her friendship, at forty-five, with three academics—one, sixty years old; the other two, thirty—and explains why their futurity differs from some progressive futurity in which she would inhabit a version of her sixty-year-old friend's life fifteen years hence and her younger colleagues would inhabit hers during the same time: "Specifically, living with advanced breast cancer, I have little chance of ever being the age my older friend is now. My friends who are thirty are equally unlikely ever to experience my present, middle age: one is living with an advanced cancer . . . the other is living with HIV. The friend who is a very healthy sixty is much the likeliest of us to be living fifteen years from now."[100] Sedgwick prefaces this description of her own and her friends' shifted futurity by noting that many never enjoy that other kind of temporality, thanks to racism, poverty, environmental toxicities. But she does not dwell there. Instead, Sedgwick sidesteps the obviously political (and for her, paranoid) reading of her friendships for a consideration of an ethics and politics that are less about exposure than animated by intimacy: "There's another sense in which [our life's narratives] slide up more intimately alongside one another than can any lives that are moving forward according to the regular schedule of the generations. It is one another immediately, one another as the present fullness of a becoming whose arc may extend no further, whom we each must learn best to apprehend, fulfill, and bear company."[101] For Sedgwick, it's not that the hermeneutic of suspicion that undergirds paranoid reading and knowledge is wrong; it's just that it leaves the reader impoverished and breathless in its wake, an aesthetic of "minimalist elegance and conceptual economy."[102] The primary impetus of paranoid reading is exposure, to leave something in full view of its nakedness, to confer power and agency to the one regarding over the one regarded. The reparative impulse, by contrast, takes what little time is left of something like a friendship of four academics whose ages span thirty years and tries to "assemble and confer plenitude on an object [such as friendship] that will then have resources to offer to an inchoate self [their individual and corporate subjectivities]."[103] Reparation gives quarter to the discrete tenderness of the affect of bounded—indeed, mortal—temporality.

Sedgwick risks the hoots and laughter of her academic colleagues by deigning to call such attention to ordinary interactions among vulnerable friends "love." She admits as much: "The vocabulary for articulating any reader's reparative motive toward a text or a culture has long been so sappy, aestheticizing, defensive, anti-intellectual, or reactionary that it's no wonder few critics are willing to describe their acquaintance with such motives."[104] But for Lin it is these acts of reading and writing reparatively, reading and writing as reparative acts, that become idealized models for managing the destructive capacities and even tendencies that psychoanalysis names as fundamental to human psyche. To treat a cultural work as tenderly as one might approach someone on her sickbed or deathbed is to render the scholarly enterprise in ways perhaps unimaginable to the current expectation of what counts as criticism, a retreat from rigor, or a disavowal of politics. Lin, however, views Sedgwickian "love" as a re-enchantment of what constitutes rigorous scholarship and trenchant politics and this form of reading as writing as a "reparative performance of love": "Affiliation with others in the same uncertain state of health led Sedgwick to the idea that companionship with the bardo of dying could produce a novel public sphere," a public organized not by rational political interests but through affective intimacies as close as the fragility of a dying body.[105] Such a public sphere would be, to cite Berlant again, a training.

Such a public sphere also mirrors Arthur Frank's citation of Albert Schweitzer's "brotherhood [*sic*] of those who bear the mark of pain."[106] Or, as Lin puts it, "The bardo of dying is a pedagogic space in which one learns from identification not only with shared disease but also with others' experience of pain and confusion. The trauma and stigma of affliction binds one to others with whom one can empathize, having in common the destabilization of one's self and world."[107] Illness teaches Sedgwick and her readers like Lin, who learn from her learning an expanded sociality that cannot assuage the losses inflicted by life-threatening or life-diminishing illness but can bear and even enjoy the company of others, "acting as a public sphere where one teaches and learns how to die, how to live, how to live on, how to accept and appreciate mortality—one's own and others, how to grieve and come to terms with loss, and how to love."[108] Such a public sphere of Sedgwick's bardo of dying is also an indefinite, unceasing learning, not only because living and dying are things worthy of being learned, but also because the very notion of reparation demands it. While she doesn't dwell on the particular Asian American inflection of the term, "reparation" is the second "r" in the decades-long campaign of "redress and reparations," the movement by

Japanese Americans and their allies to compel the U.S. government to acknowledge the ways that mass incarceration during World War II wounded, traumatized, and shattered the community, an act that continues to haunt the community generations later. The immediate effects of the success of this movement—the formal apology by the government to the Japanese American community, the pardoning of those who resisted the wartime draft, and the conferral of monetary compensation to each affected household—were the most obvious and visible expressions of the political and moral power of the campaign. But it is the final piece of reparation—the establishment of a public education fund—that commits the government indefinitely and serves to mobilize state resources to make of this form of reparation a kind of pedagogic experience from which one learns from others' affliction.[109] Such is the hope of reparation, whether a reading or writing practice or state endeavor: the forging of relationality through others' experiences of pain and confusion, the commonalities born of the destabilizations of self and world.[110]

Perhaps, then, it is not surprising that Lin's attachment to Sedgwick's writing goes far beyond the intellectually admiring and toward a kind of affection usually reserved for friends. Sentiments and sentimentality are usually hoarded as private feelings, but Lin shares them as an opening into a new public sphere: "Sedgwick's publications can function as [a 'potent, condensed, sometimes cryptic form of access to the person who would otherwise be lost']," Lin concludes her chapter, "for those of us who survive her, and who, like myself, may fall in love with a writer they have never met. . . . This Eve I have never met and yet somehow know and love has distributed parts of herself in her books and through her words. Her discourse on love enters me as part-objects with which I identify. She teaches me that publications are vital, animate, collaborative objects that perform the work of mourning and love."[111] Sedgwick beckons Lin into a sociality across time and material, the mind of Lin's organic brain touched by the inorganic animacy of the books that bear the dead scholar's name, a relationality as potent as the mercury that poisons and changes Chen's body and their relationship to the world's objects. Lin searches through Sedgwick, Lorde, and even Freud for a way to take Jain's insight—that like cancer's metastatic desire, her life has become cancer, however unwillingly—and, like Jain, takes to standing along the shores of prognostic time, watching the vast ocean of cancer's world lapping at her feet. Here she and they—all of them—stand, bearing witness to those pulled into the deep, yet not them just yet. So for now, here they are, bearing witness to the mourning and love and whatever words come to take measure of this terrible and beautiful scene.

Epilogue

Slow Time and Unprecedence

April 2020

"The model minority is not doing well," wrote Eliza Noh in 1997 under the pseudonym Lisa Park in her essay "Letter to My Sister," a haunting, eviscerating epistolary essay that explored the affective demands placed on her sibling that made life unlivable to the point of suicide for this young Asian American woman. The fragile edifice that is the performative element of every success frame narrative for Asian Americans comes undone when such impossible expectation results in what those versed in psychiatric biomedicine would call forms of mental disorder and what Noh calls more simply and accurately "living under siege." Anguish unto death isn't mental illness; it's evidence of what killed her and what is killing you and me:

Do you see what a lie it is and how it is used to reinforce the American Dream and punish those of us who don't "succeed," or who succeed "too much"? It is making me mad knowing the truth of this culture, which is so obvious and yet so strategically dissimulated in the everyday that it becomes invisible, and nothing is left but the violence that results from its disappearance. How do you point out the horror of something that is so fundamentally banal and routine that it ceases to appear traumatic? And when you do point out the lie that is the truth, you feel (and usually are) alone in seeing this and wanting to root it out. It's enough to make you paranoid, because it is such a thorough conspiracy—how can you reform something that is so structural, so absolutely essential to the constitution of this society? Therapy and social work are out of the question, because the point is not to heal or to cope—no token of change can rectify our injury. Why would you want to place yourself into the hands of an institution that seeks to resocialize you into the environment that made a mess of you in the first place? . . . Isn't our madness often the only evidence we have at all to show for this civilizing terror?[1]

Noh's essay was an early reminder that even still physically able-bodied Asian Americans have to wake up every day to face up to what's killing them, the contortions of neoliberal and model minority exemplary performance that is as psychically toxic as it is economically rewarding. Such is the cost-benefit of embodying the Asian American racial form. What the memoirs we've read together in this book gesture to in something like a utopian whisper is that there is another world that is less about better organizing, better politics, better education (though these arguably would help) than about paying attention to what breaks you and processing these feelings as a form of cultural data. And if the primary requisite to Americanness is, indeed, racism, Noh charges her parents and herself as racism's principal executioners of their daughter and her sister.

If Noh's essay insists on the horrific mess of living under siege as Asian American, the unbearability of it is that it feels impossible, like capitalism itself, to find an outside to these narratives: model minorities must reproduce until they can't anymore and they die, just as the economy must always move forward, even if we know this ship leaves so many behind, broken and dead, in its wake. To stop being this kind of Asian American or to stop living in this kind of economy seems impossible; thus, the well-meaning utopian shrugs of cultural studies in so many epilogues. Even my call to center illness as a means to imagine otherwise seems an exercise in scholarly fantasy. But, then, sometimes events happen, like the one happening as I write these concluding lines, in April 2020, in the midst of a global pandemic that introduced almost overnight terms that few people—including me—knew existed just weeks earlier: "R0 rates of infectivity"; "viral shedding"; the at-once-atomizing call to human solidarity, "social distancing." Beginning with a regional lockdown to stop it from spreading among people in China's Hubei Province during the Lunar New Year, SARS-CoV-2 novel coronavirus (COVID-19) spread quickly—exponentially. By mid-March 2020, as people began poking outside to gather in the warm weather and some college students flew to spring break to party while others, like my students, prepared for winter quarter final exams, "normal" economic activity came to an abrupt, though uneven, halt in the United States. Here, and in much of the rest of the world, "shelter-in-place" orders took effect, some with the force of law and others advisory. Suddenly the world got very quiet, at least in some places.

Reports of the novel coronavirus outbreak in Wuhan began to emerge in December 2019, but it would take another month before worries over a possible epidemic caused the World Health Organization (WHO) to call it a Public Health Emergency of International Concern. On March 11, 2020, WHO declared the global pandemic. What spread faster than the virus, at least in the initial few weeks of the outbreak, were incidents of anti-Chinese and anti-Asian rhetoric, behavior, and, sometimes, violence directed at people of Asian descent in Asian and Western countries. In late January and early February 2020, as Lunar New Year celebrations across Asia were truncated due to local and, later, national lockdowns, members of the Asian communities in places such as France, the United Kingdom, and the United States began mobilizing to challenge the racist invective directed at them for being the racial front line of public health fears. #Jenesuispasunvirus and #Iamnotavirus quickly became, pardon the metaphor, viral social media campaigns to organize diasporic Asian communities to fight off, en masse, the wave of racism that would surely increase as COVID-19 found its way into more and more places.[2] They were right: virus and violence grew exponentially throughout the winter and into the spring, which prompted Asian American scholars, activists, and policy makers to begin documenting such incidents in the United States, a sad database to remember the history that, Nayan Shah and others have reminded us, is constitutive of cultural logic. As much as Asian Americans may want to achieve with their bodies ultra-cleanliness to match their model minority social stories, their cultural washing of assimilation is a fragile prophylactic to being viewed as vectors of contagion.[3]

Given his history of deploying race throughout his campaign and administration, Donald Trump's use of the term "Chinese virus" to describe COVID-19, following his advisers' attempts to hitch the virus to a specific and necessarily different region of the world, was as predictable as it was predictably outrageous.[4] In the face of now state-sanctioned and extralegal forms of anti-Asian vulnerability making, Asian Americans responded also in predictable ways. The hopelessly improbable Asian American presidential candidate Andrew Yang, who had recently suspended his campaign, published an op-ed in the *Washington Post* on April 1, 2020, titled, "We Asian Americans Are Not the Virus, but We Can Be Part of the Cure." Yang's argument, a mediocre performance in respectability politics, comes at the essay's end: "We Asian Americans need to embrace and show our American-ness in ways we never have before." That would include literally putting on clothing that features the colors red, white, and blue (!) as a way to mitigate the shame that comes from being associated with a racially coded virus. That idea would be awfully, and obviously, reminiscent of the politics of loyalty at the heart of the Japanese American Citizens League's attempt to perform 200 percent Americanism during World War II, except that Yang himself cites the example of the 442nd Regimental Combat Team as a model for contemporary Asian America to be part of the "cure." (Of the virus? Of racism? He doesn't say.) Yang's contribution to being a "solution" for the United States is more resonant with the fantasies of Emi in John Okada's *No-No Boy*, when she chastises the despondent draft-resisting protagonist Ichiro to assert his Americanism through "make believe" and "pretend."

Asian Americanists have responded in necessary, trenchant, and predictable ways to both the vilification of Asians and Asian Americans by Trump and others who reflexively turn to white supremacy to explain most things of the world *and* Yang's model minority respectability politics. There has been no shortage of webinars, workshops, interviews, and statements from prominent Asian American activists and celebrities, as well as scholars in my field, Asian American studies, to mobilize political and intellectual resources to try to stop the spread of racist discourse and violence. On March 31, 2020, the *Journal of Asian American Studies*, the flagship publication of the Association for Asian American Studies, put out an emergency call for papers (CFP) responding to the topic "Viral Racisms: Asians/Americans and Pacific Islanders Respond to COVID-19"; the accelerated deadline for full essays to be submitted was May 1, 2020, giving scholars exactly one month to ponder an ongoing global social catastrophe. I repeat: these were all good and admirable, predictable and necessary, things. Predictability is the temporality of able-bodiedness and health. It is the measure by which one can see whether the restitution narrative (remember: tomorrow, I'll get better) still works. The threat of anti-Asian racism is the potential risk of loss of participation in temporal normality, the socially reproductive capacity for Asian Americans to live out the narratives that undergird their ability to move through the world, whether as model minorities or as deeply political creatures who are aware of that identity's deep pitfalls and have built livelihoods to critique this narrative. It remains, however, as the social warrant of this critique the right of Asian Americans to gather in time and space, in safety and health, a public schedule for cultural flourishing. Someday, when this pandemic is over, we want to be able to come together without fear that the other specter let loose—racist hate—will prevent us still from doing so. Who wouldn't want their future back?

But, hear me out: what if this future never arrives? What if COVID-19 rages on, not for weeks or months but years on end? What if we shelter in place indefinitely? How do we imagine life under quarantine, this peculiar form of living under siege? The pandemic and the governmental, social response to it, in turn, have been called unprecedented: the global reach and scale of the viral spread, its brutal mortality, and the ensuing rapidity of lockdowns across the world, however unevenly, are like nothing we've ever seen. So, too, is the "unprecedented" size of the stimulus bill rushed into law in late March 2020: $2 trillion in relief is an "unprecedented," previously unimaginable amount of money that the U.S. government socialized and is giving to corporations, small businesses, medical facilities, the unemployed, and everyday people (though, importantly, not to everyone). Unprecedented times call for unprecedented measures. But unprecedented is another word for *un*predictability, which is another word for contingency, which, as I've been trying to show, is the ontological condition of the ill body.

I am sheltering in place as I write these words to "flatten the curve," public health's metaphor to slow the spread of infection so that unchecked exponential infection rates don't overwhelm tapped-out medical workers and institutions. To help slow the rate of people falling ill from this disease, you and I, for a period of time in 2020 and maybe longer than that, had to release ourselves from the predictable and reproducible temporality that undergirded every success frame narrative of contemporary social life, the Asian American one included, and that fueled neoliberal capitalism's drive to extract value from every dimension of social life, Asian American ones included. To help save lives from very bad deaths (and they are bad because people infected with COVID-19 must, because of their infectivity, die alone and in isolation, bereft of the kindness of haptic medicine), you and I must perform the interruption and disruption of bodily immobility that are the hallmarks of the sick and disabled person. And because of this, the U.S. and global economy, which depend on mobile, able-bodied people to move through the world, has ground to an utter halt; this, in turn, has triggered unemployment in the United States that may very well exceed the joblessness of the Great Depression. As of this writing, twenty-two million people have filed for unemployment. Fewer than half of the residents of Los Angeles County still have jobs.

Here are more numbers. Before COVID-19 entered either the scientific or the popular lexicon in the United States, 4,754 persons were diagnosed with cancer every day; everyday, about 1,670 persons die from this illness.[5] More than 48,000 die from suicide every year in the United States, or about 132 per day. There are a bit fewer than 900,000 hospital beds in this country, with an average daily occupancy rate of 65 percent, or 585,000 persons spending a night in a hospital, which means that on any given day, the ill and the wounded constitute a diasporic American city roughly the size of Milwaukee, Wisconsin, or Albuquerque, New Mexico. COVID-19 has forced the "rest of us" who are, at the moment, nonresidents of these cities to interrupt our predictabilities and our mobilities, to mirror a "healthy" version of what ill bodies do every day, COVID-19's presence notwithstanding. And those of us who have suddenly found ourselves disabled by the threat of infecting others or of being infected, a kind of anticipatory illness, are at a loss as to how we live this form of life, virtual and digital forms of workplace continuity (like the remote classes and meetings I've been having) notwithstanding. Restitution narratives, buttressed by contemporary biomedicine, demand that we ask, for ourselves and for the economy, when things are going to get "better." To this I ask again: what if this "better" future never arrives?

We might, then, look to those who have dwelled a bit longer in living differential futures than most of us have, those who have developed through their pedagogies of illness a version of sick Asian Americans that doesn't equate (only) with despair and loss or, at least, holds these two feelings among a plenitude of affect. Esmé Weijun Wang's *The Collected Schizophrenias*, a series of exquisitely written essays about her life as person with schizoaffective disorder and late-stage Lyme disease, plumbs the oscillating poles of temporality that I've been pondering in this Epilogue: predictability and unprecedence, reproducibility and contingency. While at the time her work was published her mind could hold to the empirically verifiable day to day, thanks to antipsychotic medication, therapy, and intentional self-care, Wang's brain is always a hairline fracture away from getting sick again. In one chapter she describes writing a sentence while in active Cotard's delusion, the psychosis of believing that one is a corpse, about which she later wonders, "The questions instead became about percentages. What percentage of my life was going to be spent in psychosis."[6] The constant presence of her psychotic self makes the economy of the workaday impossible, so Wang's "work" as a writer must conform to her disorder's management of her time, as well as to her identity as an Asian American woman who graduated from Stanford University after Yale decided it couldn't stomach her illness, her disability too much a stain on its institutionally ableist prestige. "Who is this alleged 'person,'" Wang asks, "who is a 'person living with psychosis,' once the psychosis has set in to the point that there is nothing on the table save acceptance? When the self has been swallowed by illness, isn't it cruel to insist on a self that is not illness?"[7] Yet while she writes from the identity and subject position of a sick person, she often passes for a predictable model minority when she's out, talking about subjects such as her mental illness. At a lecture in a Chinatown clinic, presumably to help those serving other Asian Americans whose brains are versions of sick, Wang opens with her performative curriculum vitae:

> My talk for the Chinatown clinic was one that I adjusted for a variety of audiences: students, patients, doctors. It began with this line: "It was winter in my sophomore year at a prestigious university." That phrase, "prestigious university," was there to underscore my kempt hair, the silk dress, my makeup, the dignified shoes. It said, What I am about to disclose to you comes with a disclaimer. I didn't want my audience to forget that disclaimer when I began to talk about believing, for months at a time, that everyone I love is a robot. "Prestigious university" acts as a signifier of worth.[8]

Expertise in the radical unprecedence that is psychosis is wrapped in language of predictive exceptionality: Wang discloses in her memoir the fictions that Asian American speakers—and their American listeners—require to teach them what kind of life is possible if one never leaves the sickroom of our quarantines.

After her diagnosis of schizoaffective disorder, Wang received a subsequent one of Lyme disease, which explained the unpredictable bouts of searing pain that had waylaid her for months on end since 2013. In a recent essay for *New York Magazine*'s website TheCut.com, she describes what one might call a pedagogy of uncertainty that this physical illness taught her: "While in bed, riding the waves of illness, I learned to stay afloat, not knowing what was going to happen next. To live with uncertainty, even as I was suffering. And how to keep not knowing, for as long as I was alive."[9] Unlike the respectability sociality that she can play as an Asian American woman giving a lecture about her broken brain, Wang's Lyme disease undoes the predicative capacity of model minority performance. What she calls the "Illness" leaves her with radical contingency: "Not only did the symptoms *arrive* without warning, but I also feared, every time, that *this* would be the time that the pain would never back off and I would have to adapt to a new life of torture forever. During the worst, most excruciating bouts of discomfort and pain, for example, I would need to contend with the idea that it was entirely possible that I would be exactly *that sick* forever."[10] What she calls uncertainty, this contingent time, destroys all pretense of restitution, of predictive temporalities, of economies of any normative order. Illness is the enemy of inflationary pressure; it deflates and decelerates, whether you like it or not. "It seems extra cruel to make time slow down when all we want to do is get through this time faster," she writes to end the essay, "but trust me: that we will get through this very slowly is only thing of which I'm certain."[11] Illness begets slowness, stillness, stasis; some new order is in order after such chaos. But you can't hurry this new order, because illness keeps its own time.

We are all in this together. In what ways are we together in this crisis? In what ways were we so beforehand, and what affective conditions have changed that would make those of us who didn't want to belong to this call to solidarity beforehand now lean into unified action? By staying away from one another we demonstrate our togetherness, but for how long will, should, we stay away? At what point do we give up on one another and choose instead to reach for the hug, the café, the movie theater, and make one another sick beyond measure? The impulse remains, even if we know better, to want to return to the way things were so that those who consider themselves still healthy, still productive, for whom the economy still works pretty well, need not dwell on the ways that all of us are, as Mimi Khúc puts it, "differentially unwell."[12] Already, before COVID-19. So how do we get through this, however slowly? The Korean American artist Johanna Hedva pondered isolation as solidarity in the essay "Sick Woman Theory," which they begin by recounting an instance in 2014, during a bout of chronic illness that left them homebound, bedridden, and unable to join a Black Lives Matter march happening just outside their residence, except to raise a fist while horizontal. Hedva wonders aloud who else at that moment felt called to join the march but couldn't, a diaspora of sequestration that hid the larger community of allies: "I thought of all the other invisible bodies, with their fists up, tucked away and out of sight. As I lay there, unable to march, hold up a sign, shout a slogan that would be heard, or be visible in any traditional capacity as a political being, the central question of Sick Woman Theory formed: how do you throw a brick through the window of a bank if you can't get out of bed?"[13] Hedva demonstrates throughout "Sick Woman Theory" how modes, discourses, and institutions that reinforce the disabling cultures that make certain bodies sicker than others—people of color, women, queer people, differently embodied people—also render them invisible, individuate their suffering precisely so that the healthier among us can say to one another that we are in this together, but not with *them*. So to claim an identity as an Asian American, white-passing, gender-nonbinary *sick person* is also a manifesto of visibility, which is a first step to asking the question again: In what ways should we be together? Hedva writes:

> Sick Woman Theory is for those who are faced with their vulnerability and unbearable fragility, every day, and so have to fight for their

experience to be not only honored, but first made visible. For those who, in Audre Lorde's words, were never meant to survive: because this world was built against their survival. It's for my fellow spoonies, my fellow sick and crip crew. You know who you are, even if you've not been attached to a diagnosis: one of the aims of Sick Woman Theory is to resist the notion that one needs to be legitimated by an institution, so that they can try to fix you according to their terms. You don't need to be fixed, my queens—it's the world that needs the fixing. I offer this as a call to arms and a testimony of recognition. I hope that my thoughts can provide articulation and resonance, as well as tools of survival and resilience. And for those of you who are not chronically ill or disabled, Sick Woman Theory asks you to stretch your empathy this way. To face us, to listen, to see.[14]

For Hedva, the ill, disabled body is an inherent site of political protest, one's pain and suffering the signs and slogans of a dispersed public sphere. In the context of COVID-19, such insistence on this form of politics must be heightened because what chronically ill people have known, and what other vulnerable people have known—what W. E. B. DuBois once called the "second sight" that is the special vision of Black people in the United States—is that it is only in the making of one's own woundedness a site of knowledge, a data set of woundedness, that people can finally see that vulnerability, contingency, fragility, and unprecedence are the first and last instance of existence itself. Any attempt to suggest a different narrative predicated on predictive outcomes or forms of continuity are doing nothing less than engaging in endless accounts of cruel optimism, those like the American dream, the model minority, inclusive excellence. Of course, the world is shocked at the unprecedented collapse of the economy thanks to COVID-19, because it rested on the success stories of cruel optimism, those who have no problem yoking health care to their employment because those who make up this demographic, to the exclusion of so many others, were in it together, through the abandonment of others. But second sight allows us to see ourselves and others as always already differentially unwell, what Mimi Khúc tries to impart in a letter to her daughter: "I need you to understand that we are all differentially unwell, that people are vulnerable, made vulnerable, kept vulnerable. That our vulnerabilities are both our death and our life. That our vulnerabilities link us, connect us, in a web of death and survival."[15]

Hedva lies in bed and offers an invitation to you, an invitation and an insight: "The Sick Woman is anyone who does not have this guarantee of care. And crucially: the Sick Woman is who capitalism needs to perpetuate itself. . . . Because to stay alive, capitalism cannot be responsible for our care—its logic of exploitation requires that some of us die."[16] And here we arrive at the final cultural logic of restitution narratives, of which I've been saying throughout this book that Asian America's version—the model minority—has been the affective engine for all Americans' cruel optimism, and that our memoirists, physician and ill authors in their differently related ways, have sought to teach otherwise. Brought to scale, this cultural logic is the global economy now shuttered by an unprecedented, radically unpredictable, possibly terminal crisis. We are told that we must kill the economy to save lives. This is a cost too high to bear for some politicians, who thus demand a necropolitics of making explicit the expendability of some human life for the sake of capitalist immortality.

The forms of state assistance to corporations, small business, hospitals, and unemployed and employed individuals and households are unprecedented, we are told. So, too, are words now entering the public sphere that heretofore were understood as radically leftist or irrationally idealistic or fiscally irresponsible. At least for the moment, they are being considered within the rubrics of rational choice. (Rent and mortgage) forbearance, (debt) forgiveness, extended periods of (credit) grace, housing for the homeless at no cost, release of prisoners from their confinement for their and others' health: these are tender terms and instances of generosity and care that are largely absent from a system and discipline—economics—built on the epistemology of scarcity and its allocation. But I hear these words all the same on CNBC in these unprecedented times when the U.S. Congress passed in less than two weeks a fiscal giveaway of more than $2 trillion. But why $2 trillion? Why not $4 trillion? Why not $10 trillion? What is money when the need is as exponential as infection? Hedva offers a different form of exchange, in which the ill, wounded, vulnerable body is the desired political constituent and economic consumer:

> The most anti-capitalist protest is to care for another and to care for yourself. To take on the historically feminized and therefore invisible practice of nursing, nurturing, caring. To take seriously each other's vulnerability and fragility and precarity, and to support it, honor it, empower it. To protect each other, to enact and practice community. A radical kinship, an interdependent sociality, a politics of care. Because once we are all ill and confined to the bed, sharing our stories of therapies and comforts, forming support groups, bearing witness to each other's tales of trauma, prioritizing the care and love of our

sick, pained, expensive, sensitive, fantastic bodies, and there is no one left to go to work, perhaps then, finally, capitalism will screech to its much-needed, long-overdue, and motherfucking glorious halt.[17]

Here, at this nexus, Sick Woman and Marx tend to each other, as they both refuse the logic of restitution's insistence on value extraction that we are all supposed to owe, the destruction of the discipline of economics as an ethical epistemology and social organization, which is the only way that the able-bodied model minority will be forever killed, with no chance for an afterlife: "This affirmation of debt's unpayability robs debt of its calculability, of its quantifiable claim on the future earnings of worker. To be in debt forever is to refuse to balance the books, to resist paying your debt to society, and thus to throw a wrench into the very machinery of social reproduction. Think of it as a kind of irrational exuberance from below: a way of transforming default and devaluation into the very condition of possibility for radical collective politics."[18]

My meditation on speculative nonfiction asks: In your here and now, what is worth giving to imagine this place for sick people everywhere, and what is worth giving up?[19] I don't know what future this Epilogue will live in. It may very well be hopelessly dated, an expression of naïveté and stupidity. Economics is, if anything, a robust genre with many vested authors. But I write this anyway because you and I know that, before the pandemic made so much of this world unprecedented, there were many predictable things that are not worth returning to. However, when we go outside again, it is worth remembering a time when the world's aggregate demand was measured in small and great expressions of care.

Notes

INTRODUCTION

1. Julie Yip-Williams, *The Unwinding of the Miracle: A Memoir of Life, Death, and Everything That Comes After* (New York: Random House, 2019), ix.

2. Ibid., x.

3. Ibid.

4. "Best Sellers: Combined Print and E-book Nonfiction," *New York Times*, February 24, 2019, https://www.nytimes.com/books/best-sellers/2019/02/24/com bined-print-and-e-book-nonfiction/?action=click&contentCollection=Books&refer rer=https%3A%2F%2Fwww.nytimes.com%2Fbooks%2Fbest-sellers%2Fhardcover nonfiction%2F&region=Header&module=ArrowNav&version=Right&pgtype=Ref erence.

5. Julie Yip-Williams, *My Cancer Fighting Journey* (blog), https://julieyipwilliams .wordpress.com.

6. Yip-Williams, *Unwinding*, 314.

7. Tracy Smith, "Borrowed Time: Reflecting on a Life with Cancer," *CBS Sunday Morning*, March 11, 2018, https://www.cbsnews.com/news/borrowed-time -julie-yip-williams-reflecting-on-a-life-with-cancer; Richard Sandomir, "Julie Yip-Williams, Writer of Candid Blog on Cancer, Dies at 42," *New York Times*, March 22, 2018, https://www.nytimes.com/2018/03/22/obituaries/julie-yip-williams-dies -writer-of-candid-blog-on-cancer.html.

8. Ellen D. Wu, *The Color of Success: Asian Americans and the Origins of the Model Minority* (Princeton, NJ: Princeton University Press, 2013); Madeline Y. Hsu, *The Good Immigrants: How the Yellow Peril Became the Model Minority* (Prince-

ton, NJ: Princeton University Press, 2015); Jennifer Lee and Min Zhou, *The Asian American Achievement Paradox* (New York: Russell Sage Foundation, 2015).

9. Keith Osajima, "Asian Americans as the Model Minority: An Analysis of the Popular Press Image in the 1960s and 1980s," in *Reflections on Shattered Windows: Promises and Prospects for Asian American Studies*, edited by Gary Okihiro (Pullman: Washington State University Press, 1988), 165–174.

In the wake of the murder of George Floyd and the ensuing protests that insisted that #blacklivesmatter, Viet Thanh Nguyen contributed an article to a special issue of *Time* magazine in which he reintroduced the concept of the model minority to a general readership, wedging in the Asian Americanist critique by writing, "This is what it means to be a model minority: to be invisible in most circumstances because we are doing what we are supposed to be doing, like my parents, until we become hypervisible because we are doing what we do too well, like the Korean shopkeepers [during the Los Angeles Uprisings of 1992]. Then the model minority becomes the Asian invasion, and the Asian-American model minority, which had served to prove the success of capitalism, bears the blame when capitalism fails": Viet Thanh Nguyen, "Asian Americans Are Still Caught in the Trap of the 'Model Minority' Stereotype, and It Creates Inequality for All," *Time*, July 6, 2020, https://time.com/5859206/anti-asian-racism-america. But what is more durable, more pernicious, and less acknowledged in his account are the affective attachments that Asian Americans themselves hold to model minority discourse as a life practice, one as cellular to social life as the anti-Blackness called out by the protests in 2020.

10. Such is the demand of the "success frame" that Lee and Zhou identify as the achievement paradox of Asian Americans: Lee and Zhou, *Asian American Achievement Paradox*. It is a paradox because such social valorization mitigates what Claire Jean Kim argues is the structural "civic ostracism" that Asian Americans historically have suffered. It is this countervailing force, between the valuation of their educational and economic attainment and their durable outsiderness, that triangulates their position vis-à-vis normative whiteness and the devaluation of Black people in the United States: Claire Jean Kim, "The Racial Triangulation of Asian Americans," *Politics and Society* 27, no. 1 (1999): 105–138.

11. Writes Matthew Teague in a review of Yip-Williams's memoir, "She offers an implicit challenge, then, to the rest of us. We may not be able to mark the moment of our deaths on a calendar, but it waits there nonetheless. So we should, by her *model*, live even as we are dying": Matthew Teague, "*The Unwinding of the Miracle* Review: Cancer Memoir is an Epic in Miniature," *The Guardian*, February 17, 2019, https://www.theguardian.com/books/2019/feb/17/the-unwinding-of-the -miracle-review-cancer-memoir-julie-yip-williams, emphasis added.

12. Lee and Zhou, *Asian American Achievement Paradox*, 14–16.

13. Angela Duckworth, *Grit: The Power of Passion and Perseverance*, TED Talks Education, April 2013, video and transcript, https://www.ted.com/talks

/angela_lee_duckworth_grit_the_power_of_passion_and_perseverance; Angela Duckworth, *Grit: The Power of Passion and Perseverance* (New York: Scribner, 2016), 8.

14. Here Duckworth internalizes what earlier sociologists have identified as a cardinal characteristic of contemporary Asian American self-perceptions filtered through a model minority lens: Paul Wong, Chienping Faith Lai, Richard Nagasawa, and Tieming Lin, "Asian Americans as a Model Minority: Self-Perceptions and Perceptions by Other Racial Groups," *Sociological Perspectives* 41, no. 1 (1998): 95–118.

15. Duckworth, *Grit*, 271. This is actually the penultimate story of the book's conclusion. Duckworth's final example is the author and journalist Ta-Nehisi Coates upon the publication of his memoir, *Between the World and Me*, and his selection as a fellow MacArthur "genius" in 2015. Attributing Coates's newfound fame to the grit he exhibited through the stresses of writing and unemployment, Duckworth makes only passing reference to his growing up with experiences of precarity; the deep precarity of Black life in the United States, of course, occupies and thematizes much of his book. Anti-Black racism, the book's final sentence suggests, meets its end if one can work "toward excellence": ibid., 277.

16. Ibid, xv, emphasis added.

17. Hisaye Yamamoto, "Las Vegas Charley," in *Seventeen Syllables and Other Stories* (New Brunswick, NJ: Rutgers University Press, 2001), 70–85; Ronyoung Kim, *Clay Walls* (Sag Harbor, NY: Permanent, 1987).

18. Douglas Baynton, "Disability and the Justification of Inequality in American History," in *The New Disability History: American Perspectives*, edited by Paul Longmore and Lauri Umansky (New York: New York University Press, 2001), 33–57.

19. "This common strategy for attaining equal rights, which seeks to distance one's own group from imputations of disability and therefore tacitly accepts the idea that disability is a legitimate reason for inequality, is perhaps one of the factors responsible for making discrimination against people with disabilities so persistent and the struggle for disability rights so difficult": Baynton, "Disability," 51.

20. Tobin Siebers, "Disability in Theory: From Social Constructionism to the New Realism of the Body," in *The Disability Studies Reader*, 2d ed., edited by Lennard J. Davis (New York: Routledge, 2006), 181.

21. Eli Clare, *Brilliant Imperfection: Grappling with Cure* (Durham, NC: Duke University Press, 2017); Eunjung Kim, *Curative Violence: Rehabilitating Disability, Gender, and Sexuality in Modern Korea* (Durham, NC: Duke University Press, 2017).

22. G. Thomas Couser, *Signifying Bodies: Disability in Contemporary Life Writing* (Ann Arbor: University of Michigan Press, 2009), 3.

23. Katherine Mack and Jonathan Alexander, "The Ethics of Memoir: *Ethos* in Uptake," *Rhetoric Society Quarterly* 49, no. 1 (2019): 49–70.

24. Tobin Siebers, *Disability Theory* (Ann Arbor: University of Michigan Press, 2008); Arthur Frank, *The Wounded Storyteller: Body, Illness, and Ethics* (Chicago: University of Chicago Press, 1995); Rita Charon, *Narrative Medicine: Honoring the Stories of Illness* (New York: Oxford University Press, 2008).

25. Asian Americans are, however, blogging about their experiences of illness and other forms of wounded embodiment. I write about some of them in Chapter 3.

26. Sucheng Chan, "You're Short, Besides!" in *Making Waves: An Anthology of Writings by and about Asian American Women*, edited by Diane Yen-Mai Wong and Asian Women United of California (Boston: Beacon, 1989), 266.

27. Irmo Marini, "Cross-Cultural Counseling Issues of Males Who Sustain a Disability," *The Psychological and Social Impact of Illness and Disability*, 6th ed., edited by Irmo Marini and Mark Stebnicki (New York: Springer, 2012), 153.

28. erin Khuê Ninh, *Ingratitude: The Debt-Bound Daughter in Asian American Literature* (New York: New York University Press, 2009), 11.

29. This possessive investment in optimizing an Asian American *bios* (à la Giorgio Agamben) to secure model minority formation helps to answer Rachel Lee's provocative question that forms both her argument and method. She writes, "Given that race has been acknowledged not as biological but as a discursive (legal-juridical) construction and as an outgrowth of historically variable political-economic formations, how is it then that Asian American artists, authors, and performers keep scrutinizing their body parts?": Rachel C. Lee, *The Exquisite Corpse of Asian America: Biopolitics, Biosociality, and Posthuman Ecologies* (New York: New York University Press, 2014), 10. Bodies matter to upholding Asian American ableisms and are often the first level of interrogation.

30. "Diversity in Medicine: Facts and Figures 2019," Association of American Medical Colleges website, n.d., https://www.aamc.org/data-reports/workforce/re port/diversity-medicine-facts-and-figures-2019.

31. Michelle Au, *This Won't Hurt a Bit (and Other White Lies): My Education in Medicine and Motherhood* (New York: Grand Central, 2011), 309; Anthony Youn with Alan Eisenstock, *In Stitches: A Memoir* (New York: Gallery, 2011).

32. Fitzhugh Mullan, "The Metrics of the Physician Brain Drain," *New England Journal of Medicine* 353 (2005):1810–1818.

33. "Diversity in Medicine."

34. Atul Gawande, *Being Mortal: Medicine and What Matters in the End* (New York: Metropolitan, 2014); Fionnuala McHugh, "How Doctors Fail the Dying, by *Being Mortal* Author Atul Gawande," *South China Morning Post*, January 1, 2016, https://www.scmp.com/magazines/post-magazine/books/article/1896501/how -doctors-fail-dying-being-mortal-author-atul; Tom Jennings, prod., "Being Mortal," *Frontline*, broadcast February 10, 2015, https://www.pbs.org/wgbh/frontline /film/being-mortal.

35. Gawande remained as the chair of Haven's board even after he stepped down as its chief executive: Casey Ross and Erin Brodwin, "Atul Gawande to Depart as

CEO of Health Venture, Haven," *Boston Globe*, May 12, 2020, https://www.bos tonglobe.com/2020/05/12/business/atul-gawande-depart-ceo-health-venture-hav en. Less than a year later, the entire venture folded in failure. "Amazon, Berkshire Hathaway And JP Morgan Health Care Partnership Fails," National Public Radio, January 5, 2021, https://www.npr.org/2021/01/05/953653380/amazon-berkshire -hathaway-and-jp-morgan-health-care-partnership-fails.

36. Siddhartha Mukherjee, *The Emperor of All Maladies: A Biography of Cancer* (New York: Scribner, 2010); Ken Burns, dir., *Cancer: The Emperor of All Maladies*, film, PBS, March 30, 2015, https://www.pbs.org/show/story-cancer-emperor-all -maladies.

37. Siddhartha Mukherjee, *Gene: An Intimate History* (New York: Scribner, 2016).

38. Abraham Verghese, "A Doctor's Touch," TEDGlobal 2011, video and tran-script, https://www.ted.com/talks/abraham_verghese_a_doctor_s_touch.

39. "About Vivek," Dr. Vivek H. Murthy website, https://www.vivekmurthy .com/about.

40. Paul Kalanithi, *When Breath Becomes Air* (New York: Random House, 2016).

41. Prabhjot Singh, *Dying and Living in the Neighborhood: A Street-Level View of America's Healthcare Promise* (Baltimore: Johns Hopkins University Press, 2016).

42. Tara Fickle, *The Race Card: From Gaming Technologies to Model Minorities* (New York: New York University Press, 2019), 97.

43. Jeffrey P. Bishop, *The Anticipatory Corpse: Medicine, Power, and the Care of the Dying* (South Bend, IN: Notre Dame University Press, 2011), 18.

44. "Curative violence occurs when cure is what actually frames the presence of disability as a problem and ends up destroying the subject in the curative process. . . . The violence associated with cure exists at two levels: first, the violence of denying a place for disability and illness as different ways of living and, second, the physical and material violence against people with disabilities that are justified in the name of cure": Kim, *Curative Violence*, 14.

45. Frank, *Wounded Storyteller*, 55.

46. Fred Ho, *Diary of a Radical Cancer Warrior: Fighting Cancer and Capital-ism at the Cellular Level* (New York: Skyhorse, 2011), 175.

47. Frank, *Wounded Storyteller*, 114.

48. Brandy Liên Worrall, *What Doesn't Kill Us* (Vancouver: Rabbit Fool, 2014).

49. Keith Wailoo, *How Cancer Crossed the Color Line* (New York: Oxford University Press, 2011), 15.

50. Ibid., 179.

51. Lauren Berlant, *The Female Complaint: The Unfinished Business of Senti-mentality in American Culture* (Durham, NC: Duke University Press, 2008), 21.

52. Christine Hyung-Oak Lee, *Tell Me Everything You Don't Remember: The Stroke That Changed My Life* (New York: Ecco, 2017).

53. Ibid., 247.

54. Jane Danielewicz, *Contemporary Memoirs in Action: How to Do Things with Memoir* (New York: Palgrave Macmillan, 2018), 1.

55. Ibid.

56. William Cheng, *Just Vibrations: The Purpose of Sounding Good* (Ann Arbor: University of Michigan Press, 2016), 7.

57. Nodding to Arthur Frank, *Letting Stories Breathe: A Socio-Narratology* (Chicago: University of Chicago Press, 2010).

CHAPTER 1

1. Jhumpa Lahiri, *The Namesake* (New York: Houghton Mifflin, 2003), 135, emphasis added.

2. Min Hyoung Song, *The Children of 1965: On Writing, and Not Writing, as an Asian American* (Durham, NC: Duke University Press, 2013), 345.

3. Lavina Dhingra and Floyd Cheung, eds., *Naming Jhumpa Lahiri: Canons and Controversies* (Lanham, MD: Lexington, 2012), xx.

4. Ibid.

5. Ibid.

6. Jhumpa Lahiri, "Teach Yourself Italian," *New Yorker*, vol. 91, no. 39, December 7, 2015, 30–36, https://www.newyorker.com/magazine/2015/12/07/teach-yourself-italian; Jhumpa Lahiri, *In Other Words*, trans. Ann Goldstein (New York: Knopf, 2016).

7. Lahiri, "Teach Yourself Italian," 35.

8. Min Hyoung Song, "The Children of 1965: Allegory, Postmodernism, and Jhumpa Lahiri's *The Namesake*," *Twentieth-Century Literature* 53, no. 3 (Fall 2007): 355.

9. Lahiri, "Teach Yourself Italian," 34.

10. Mark McGurl, *The Program Era: Postwar Fiction and the Rise of Creative Writing* (Cambridge, MA: Harvard University Press, 2011), 34.

11. Sanjoy Chakravorty, Devesh Kapur, and Nirvikar Singh, *The Other One Percent: Indians in America* (New York: Oxford University Press, 2017), 24.

12. Ibid., 62.

13. Eram Alam, "Cold War Crises: Foreign Medical Graduates Respond to U.S. Doctor Shortages, 1965–1975," *Social History of Medicine* (March 2018): 1–20.

14. Alam notes also that "occupational closure was not only a practice for managing economic and professional aspects of medicine; it was also an exclusionary social strategy aimed at cultivating a specific physician image": ibid., 7. She highlights the ways that the American Medical Association helped to standardize medical education, credentialing, and other practices, especially in the first half of the twentieth century, to turn U.S. medicine into the elite, white, and male

profession that it became by the time the question of turning to foreign physicians became a national question.

15. Ibid., 16.

16. Ibid.

17. Chakravorty et al., *Other One Percent*, 29.

18. Alam, "Cold War Crises," 20.

19. Padma Rangaswamy, *Namasté America: Indian Immigrants in an American Metropolis* (University Park: Pennsylvania State University Press, 2000), 58–59.

20. Jane Iwamura, *Virtual Orientalism: Asian Religions and American Popular Culture* (New York: Oxford University Press, 2011), 79.

21. Ibid., 87–90.

22. Eram Alam, "The Care of Foreigners: A History of South Asian Physicians in the United States, 1965–2016" (Ph.D. diss., University of Pennsylvania, Philadelphia, 2016), 222.

23. Vijay Prashad, *The Karma of Brown Folk* (Minneapolis: University of Minnesota Press, 2000), 58.

24. Ibid., 66–67.

25. Ibid., 53.

26. Ibid., 56–57.

27. Deepak Chopra, *Ageless Body, Timeless Mind: The Quantum Alternative to Growing Old* (New York: Harmony, 1993), 24.

28. Sarah Benet-Weiser, *AuthenticTM: The Politics of Ambivalence in a Brand Culture* (New York: New York University Press, 2012), 192–197; Iwamura, *Virtual Orientalism*, 108–110; Gordon Pennycook, James Allan Cheyne, Nathaniel Barr, Derek J. Koehler, and Jonathan A. Fugelsang, "On the Reception and Deception of Pseudo-Profound Bullshit," *Judgment and Decision Making* 10, no. 6 (November 2015): 549–563; Robert Barnett and Cathy Sears, "JAMA Gets Into an Indian Herbal Jam," *Science*, vol. 254, October 11, 1991, 188–189; Valerie Strauss, "Scientist: Why Deepak Chopra Is Driving Me Crazy," *Washington Post*, May 15, 2015, https://www.washingtonpost.com/news/answer-sheet/wp/2015/05/15/scientist-why-deepak-chopra-is-driving-me-crazy.

29. Iwamura, *Virtual Orientalism*, 20.

30. Gupta attended and graduated from the University of Michigan Medical School in 1993 and serves on the medical faculty at Emory University, in addition to his positions at Grady Memorial and CNN.

31. These two physical modalities—Gupta facing the camera bestowing medical knowledge; Gupta in motion performing and transmitting his medical skill—are visual reminders of the biopolitical discipline expected of physicians to assert authority in clinical and discursive spaces, to make audiences and potential patients receptive listeners. Writes the medical anthropologist Rachel Prentice, "Medical education reworks the trainee's body and being. Over the years, trainees become professionals who are prepared to bear the profound responsibility for

treating others": Rachel Prentice, *Bodies in Formation: An Ethnography of Anatomy and Surgery Education* (Durham, NC: Duke University Press, 2013), 3.

32. Arthur Frank, *The Wounded Storyteller: Body, Illness, and Ethics* (Chicago: University of Chicago Press, 1995), 6.

33. Sanjay Gupta, *Cheating Death: The Doctors and Medical Miracles That Are Saving Lives against All Odds* (New York: Grand Central Life and Style, 2009), xvi.

34. Ibid., 365.

35. Ibid., 49.

36. Disability activism and, later, its academic study have been central to the dismantling of medical hegemony over the body's epistemology. "To move from the passive position of the silenced object of discourse in the cultural locations of disability to the active position of producer of knowledge about the social, political, and phenomenological aspects of disability ability destabilizes any number of objectifying practices. This change alone will prove monumental not because people with disabilities inherently know the truth of their own social and biological lives, but rather because their visible entry into the discourse of their bodies makes all speaking positions in the field shift, becoming necessarily self-conscious and increasingly self-reflexive": Sharon L. Snyder and David T. Mitchell, *Cultural Locations of Disability* (Chicago: University of Chicago Press, 2005), 203. The term "bodymind" is from Margaret Price, "The Bodymind Problem and the Possibilities of Pain," *Hypatia* 30, no. 1 (Winter 2015): 268–284.

37. Abraham Verghese, *My Own Country: A Doctor's Story of a Town and Its People in the Age of Aids* (New York: Simon and Schuster, 1994), 17.

38. Ibid., 22.

39. Ibid.

40. Quoted in Cynthia Wu, *Chang and Eng Reconnected: The Original Siamese Twins in American Culture* (Philadelphia: Temple University Press, 2012), 111.

41. Jay Timothy Dolmage, *Disabled upon Arrival: Eugenics, Immigration, and the Construction of Race and Disability* (Columbus: Ohio State University Press, 2018), 4–5.

42. "Between 1966 and 1977, of the Indian Americans who migrated to the United States, 83 percent entered under the occupational category of professional and technical workers (roughly 20,000 scientists with Ph.D.'s, 40,000 engineers, and 25,000 doctors)": Prashad, *Karma*, 75.

43. Tobin Siebers, *Disability Theory* (Ann Arbor: University of Michigan Press, 2008), 8.

44. Ibid., 9.

45. Ibid., 8.

46. What has remained consistent in immigration policy, even part of the 1965 act, is the ability to deny entry or adjust the status of a resident based on her or his risk of becoming a "public charge." One's seeming dependence on the government for subsistence is grounds to bar her entry: see U.S. Citizenship and Immigration

Services, "Green Card: Public Charge Alert," March 19, 2021, https://www.uscis.gov/greencard/public-charge.

47. Verghese, *My Own Country*, 22.

48. Ibid., 80–81.

49. Rajini Srikanth, "Ethnic Outsider as the Ultimate Insider: The Paradox of Verghese's 'My Own Country,'" *MELUS* 29, nos. 3–4 (Autumn–Winter 2004): 436–437.

50. Verghese, *My Own Country*, 126.

51. Christopher T. Fan, "Melancholy Transcendence: Ted Chiang and Asian American Postracial Form," *Post45* (November 2014), http://post45.research.yale.edu/2014/11/melancholy-transcendence-ted-chiang-and-asian-american-postracial-form.

52. Margalit Fox, "They Were Aliens in That Town," *New York Times*, August 28, 1994, 380.

53. Suzanne Poirier, *Doctors in the Making: Memoirs and Medical Education*, Kindle ed. (Iowa City: University of Iowa Press, 2009).

54. Ella Kusnetz provides an example of this mode of anti-Sacks criticism, writing, "So what, finally, is the Sacks phenomenon really all about? Not much more than an outsized ambition which has prompted him to present himself in all his books as the very model of the wise and sensitive healer—the hero of modern medicine—and that image of him has caught on, with everyone from Anatole Broyard to the executives at Columbia Pictures": Ella Kusnetz, "The Soul of Oliver Sacks," *The Massachusetts Review* 33, no. 2 (Summer 1992), 197.

55. William Howarth, "Oliver Sacks: The Ecology of Writing Science," *Modern Language Studies* 20, no. 4 (Autumn 1990), 104–105.

56. "In medicine," the Sacks scholar Andrew John Hall explains, "Romantic Science sought to construct a rigorous, authoritative, but also empathetic, therapeutic discourse about human beings and their experiences: a science that was not atomistically reductionist, but embodied the 'richness' and 'the wealth of living reality'": Andrew John Hull, "Fictional Father? Oliver Sacks and the Revalidation of Pathography," *Medical Humanities* 39 (2013): 109.

57. "The eye of science does not probe a 'thing' an event isolated from other things or events. Its real object is to see and understand the way a thing or event relates to other things or events . . . to ascertain a network of important relations (and it) . . . accomplishes the classical aim of explaining facts, while not losing sight of the romantic aim of preserving the manifold richness of the subject": ibid., 109.

58. Oliver Sacks, *An Anthropologist on Mars: Seven Paradoxical Tales* (New York: Knopf, 1995), 250.

59. Ibid., 267.

60. Ibid.

61. "An Introduction to *The New Yorker*," in *Twentieth-Century Literary Criticism*, vol. 58, edited by Jennifer Gariepy (Detroit: Gale, 1995), http://link.gale

group.com/apps/doc/GOLOCV654144738/LCO?u=univca20&sid=LCO&xid=c 30a3b78.

62. György Lukács, *Soul and Form*, edited by John T. Sanders and Katie Terazakis, translated by Anna Bostock (New York: Columbia University Press, 2010), 18.

63. Theodor Adorno, "The Essay as Form," *New German Critique* no. 32 (Spring–Summer 1984): 151–171.

64. Elena Gualtieri, "The Essay as Form: Virginia Woolf and the Literary Tradition," *Textual Practice* 12, no. 1 (1998): 50.

65. Fiona Green, "Elizabeth Bishop in Brazil and the *New Yorker*," *Journal of American Studies* 46, no. 4 (2012): 805.

66. Atul Gawande, "No Mistake," *New Yorker*, March 30, 1998, 76.

67. Ibid., 81.

68. Ira Byock, *Dying Well: The Prospect for Growth at the End of Life* (New York: Riverhead, 1997); Sherwin Nuland, *How We Die: Reflections on Life's Final Chapter* (New York: Knopf, 1994).

69. Atul Gawande, "Letting Go," *New Yorker*, August 2, 2010, https://www.newyorker.com/magazine/2010/08/02/letting-go-2. This essay was reprinted with minimal editing in Atul Gawande, *Being Mortal: Medicine and What Matters in the End* (New York: Metropolitan, 2014). Subsequent references to this essay are from the book version.

70. Gawande, *Being Mortal*, 150.

71. Ibid., 152.

72. Ibid.

73. This is categorically different from the ways that "quality of life" discourses are mobilized to truncate or even deny services to disabled people or use ableist notions of health and "quality of life" to engage in what disability studies scholars call the "new eugenics," which seeks to abort fetuses that bear markings of congenital disability: see Adrienne Asch, "Recognizing Death while Affirming Life: Can End of Life Reform Uphold a Disabled Person's Interest in Continued Life?" *Hastings Center Report* 35, no. 6 (November–December 2005): S31–S36; Ivan Brown, Roy I. Brown, and Alice Schippers, "A Quality of Life Perspective on the New Eugenics," *Journal of Policy and Practice in Intellectual Disabilities* 16, no. 2 (June 2019): 121–126.

74. Gawande, *Being Mortal*, 172, 189.

75. Ibid., 153, 173.

76. Ibid., 169.

77. Tom Jennings, prod., "Being Mortal," *Frontline*, broadcast February 10, 2015, https://www.pbs.org/wgbh/frontline/film/being-mortal.

78. Gawande, *Being Mortal*, 169.

79. Lisa Diedrich, *Treatments: Language, Politics, and the Culture of Illness* (Minneapolis: University of Minnesota Press, 2007), 150–151.

80. Diedrich, *Treatments*, 157.

81. Gawande, *Being Mortal*, 171–172.

82. Ibid., 188.

83. Rita Charon, *Narrative Medicine: Honoring the Stories of Illness* (New York: Oxford University Press, 2008), 131–132.

84. Adorno, "Essay as Form," 171.

85. Atul Gawande, "Big Med," *New Yorker*, August 13, 2012, https://www.new yorker.com/magazine/2012/08/13/big-med.

86. Gawande, *Being Mortal*, 212–213.

87. Ibid., 218.

88. Ibid.

89. Ibid., 258.

90. Ibid., 259.

91. Verghese, *My Own Country*, 424.

92. Sunita Puri, *That Good Night: Life and Medicine in the Eleventh Hour* (New York: Viking, 2019), 11.

93. Ibid., 113.

94. Ibid., 118.

CHAPTER 2

1. Nora Gallagher, *Moonlight Sonata at the Mayo Clinic* (New York: Vintage, 2014), 24.

2. G. Thomas Couser, *Signifying Bodies: Disability in Contemporary Life Writing* (Ann Arbor: University of Michigan Press, 2009), 3.

3. Arthur Frank, *The Wounded Storyteller: Body, Illness, and Ethics* (Chicago: University of Chicago Press, 1995), 18.

4. "Figure 18: Percentage of All Active Physicians by Race/Ethnicity, 2018," *Diversity in Medicine: Facts and Figures 2019*, Association of American Medical Colleges website, n.d., https://www.aamc.org/data-reports/workforce/interactive-data /figure-18-percentage-all-active-physicians-race/ethnicity-2018.

5. Danielle Ofri, *What Patients Say, What Doctors Hear* (New York: Beacon, 2017).

6. Sunita Puri, *That Good Night: Life and Medicine in the Eleventh Hour* (New York: Viking, 2019), 291.

7. Virginia Held, *The Ethics of Care: Personal, Political, and Global* (New York: Oxford University Press, 2007).

8. Rosemarie Garland-Thomson, "Integrating Disability, Transforming Feminist Theory," *NWSA Journal* 14, no. 3 (Autumn 2002): 1–32.

9. James Kyung-Jin Lee, "Elegies of Social Life: The Wounded Asian American," *Journal of Race, Ethnicity, and Religion* 3, no. 2.7 (January 2012): 1–21.

10. Suzanne Poirier, *Doctors in the Making: Memoirs and Medical Education*, Kindle ed. (Iowa City: University of Iowa Press, 2009), loc. 635–636.

11. Ibid., loc. 1042–1044.

12. Oliver Sacks, *On the Move: A Life* (New York: Knopf, 2015).

13. Damon Tweedy, *Black Man in a White Coat* (New York: Picador, 2015).

14. Michelle Au, *This Won't Hurt a Bit (and Other White Lies): My Education in Medicine and Motherhood* (New York: Grand Central, 2011), 24.

15. Ibid., 26.

16. Ibid., 26–27.

17. Rita Charon, *Narrative Medicine: Honoring the Stories of Illness* (New York: Oxford University Press, 2008), 19.

18. Ibid., 21.

19. Poirier, *Doctors*, loc. 264–265.

20. Ibid., loc. 651.

21. Frank, *Wounded Storyteller*, 81.

22. Poirier, *Doctors*, loc. 662–663.

23. Pauline Chen, *Final Exam: A Surgeon's Reflections on Mortality* (New York: Knopf, 2007), 17.

24. Ibid., 45.

25. Au, *This Won't Hurt*, 33, 34.

26. Ibid., 34.

27. Michel Foucault, *The Birth of the Clinic*, translated by Alan Sheridan Smith (New York: Pantheon, 1973), 115.

28. Au, *This Won't Hurt*, 4.

29. Foucault, *Clinic*, 8.

30. Au, *This Won't Hurt*, 122.

31. Ibid., 129.

32. Ibid., 85.

33. Ibid., 90–91.

34. Ibid., 91–92.

35. Michelle Young, *What Patients Taught Me: A Medical Student's Journey* (Seattle: Sasquatch, 2007), x.

36. Ibid., 12.

37. Ibid., 29.

38. Ibid., 29.

39. Ibid., 81.

40. Ibid., 115.

41. Ann Jurecic, *Illness as Narrative* (Pittsburgh: University of Pittsburgh Press, 2012), 11.

42. Ibid., 14.

43. Young, *Patients*, 116.

44. *Touching Feeling: Affect, Pedagogy, Performativity* was Sedgwick's final book, and she wrote many of the essays that make up the book over the course of the very same years that she lived with and was treated for cancer: Eve Kosofsky

Sedgwick, *Touching Feeling: Affect, Pedagogy, Performativity* (Durham, NC: Duke University Press, 2003).

45. Ibid., 8.

46. Sedgwick's critical regard of "paranoid reading" and her development of "reparative reading" have helped usher in modes of criticism that are also worried about the preponderance, even dominance, of critique as a principal ethic and political impulse. Literary critics such as Rita Felski and social scientists such as Bruno Latour have put forth in their respective fields a "postcritique" mode of reading and inquiry that seeks to learn "to be affected by the lives of others." In response, scholars such as Bruce Robbins argue that postcritique runs the risk of "political quietism," noting especially that "the post-critiquers have dislodged and disrespected the experience of African Americans, for whom paranoia is a perfectly acceptable language for the experience of systemic racial injustice." Robbins does note that Sedgwick herself never dismissed paranoid reading as an incorrect practice, but one that perhaps could have found, through a "beside" posture, a balance. Of course, emergent fields such as gender, queer, and ethnic studies have always mobilized the array of critical consideration, as the care of bodies wounded by systemic injustices are as important as the uncovering of structures of oppression. See Rita Felski, *The Limits of Critique* (Chicago: University of Chicago Press, 2015); Bruno Latour, "Why Has Critique Run Out of Steam? From Matters of Fact to Matters of Concern," *Critical Inquiry* 30 (2004): 225–248; Bruce Robbins, "Not So Well Attached," *PMLA* 132, no. 2 (2017): 371–376; Bruce Robbins, "Reading Bad," *Los Angeles Review of Books*, January 21, 2018, https://lareviewofbooks.org /article/reading-bad; Elizabeth S. Anker and Rita Felski, eds., *Critique and Postcritique* (Durham, NC: Duke University Press, 2017).

47. Sedgwick, *Touching Feeling*, 8.

48. Ibid., 149.

49. Craig Irvine, "The Other Side of Silence: Levinas, Medicine, and Literature," *Literature and Medicine* 24, no. 1 (February 2005): 13.

50. Ibid., 14.

51. Ibid., 15.

52. Sandeep Jauhar, *Intern: A Doctor's Initiation* (New York: Farrar, Straus, and Giroux, 2007), 40.

53. Ibid., 69.

54. Ibid.

55. Ibid., 11.

56. Ibid.

57. Ibid., 160.

58. Charon, *Narrative Medicine*, 87, 89.

59. Jauhar, *Intern*, 143.

60. Ibid., 181.

61. Ibid., 286.

62. Ibid., 289.

63. It has also turned him into the kind of South Asian male medical authority that we see in Chapter 1. Jauhar continues to write a regular column in the *New York Times* as one of the newspaper's main medical correspondents.

64. Chen, *Final Exam*, 5.

65. Ibid., 48–49.

66. Ibid., 49.

67. Ibid., 53.

68. Ibid., 54.

69. Ibid., 88.

70. Lauren Berlant, *The Female Complaint: The Unfinished Business of Sentimentality in American Culture* (Durham, NC: Duke University Press, 2008), 5.

71. "N[ational] H[ealth] E[xpenditure] Fact Sheet: Historical NHE, 2019," Centers for Medicare and Medicaid Services website, n.d., https://www.cms.gov /Research-Statistics-Data-and-Systems/Statistics-Trends-and-Reports/National HealthExpendData/NHE-Fact-Sheet.

72. Lauren Berlant, *Cruel Optimism* (Durham, NC: Duke University Press, 2011), 24.

73. Chen, *Final Exam*, 78.

74. Ibid., 179.

75. Ibid., 134.

76. Ibid., 173.

77. Ibid., 174.

78. Ibid., 175.

79. Ibid., 180.

80. Ibid., 98.

81. Ibid., 99.

82. In an address delivered at the University of California, Irvine, in October 2019, Chen discussed how physicians deliberately use the passive voice to obfuscate responsibility, to achieve through language the gulf that separates them from their patients' suffering: Pauline Chen, "Swimming the Sea: A Surgeon on Suffering," video, posted by University of California, Irvine, Humanities Center, November 5, 2019, https://www.youtube.com/watch?v=K9rvMhgFegU.

83. Chen, *Final Exam*, 100.

84. Ibid., 101.

85. Ibid., 126.

86. Ibid., 126–127.

87. Ibid., 127.

88. Ibid., 129.

89. Ibid., 139.

90. Ibid., 199–200.

91. Ibid., 201.

92. Ibid., 203.

93. Ibid., 211.

94. Ibid., 218.

95. Charon, *Narrative Medicine*, 181.

CHAPTER 3

1. Paul Kalanithi, *When Breath Becomes Air* (New York: Random House, 2016), 116.

2. Ibid., 105.

3. Ibid., 120.

4. Arthur Frank, *The Wounded Storyteller: Body, Illness, and Ethics* (Chicago: University of Chicago Press, 1995), 56.

5. Ibid., 77.

6. Kalanithi, *Breath*, 120.

7. Paul Costello, "Five Years Later: Lucy Kalanithi on Loss, Grief and Love," *Scope* (blog), April 20, 2020, https://scopeblog.stanford.edu/2020/04/20/five-years-later-lucy-kalanithi-on-loss-grief-and-love.

8. Nora Krug, "'When Breath Becomes Air': Young Doctor's Last Words of Wisdom, Hope," *Washington Post*, January 8, 2016, https://www.washingtonpost.com/entertainment/books/when-breath-becomes-air-in-a-young-doctors-final-words-wisdom-and-hope/2016/01/08/aa5a8402-b60e-11e5-9388-466021d971de_story.html.

9. Henry Marsh, "*When Breath Becomes Air* by Paul Kalanithi—Review: Thoughtful and Poignant," *Guardian*, January 31, 2016, https://www.theguardian.com/books/2016/jan/31/when-breath-becomes-air-paul-kalanithi-review.

10. Anne Hunsaker Hawkins, *Reconstructing Illness: Studies in Pathography* (West Lafayette, IN: Purdue University Press, 1998).

11. Fred Ho, *Diary of a Radical Cancer Warrior: Fighting Cancer and Capitalism at the Cellular Level* (New York: Skyhorse, 2011).

12. Brandy Liên Worrall, *What Doesn't Kill Us* (Vancouver: Rabbit Fool, 2014).

13. Padma Lakshmi, *Love, Loss, and What We Ate: A Memoir* (New York: Ecco, 2016).

14. Christine Hyung-Oak Lee, *Tell Me Everything You Don't Remember: The Stroke That Changed My Life* (New York: Ecco, 2017).

15. Esmé Weijun Wang, *The Collected Schizophrenias: Essays* (Minneapolis: Graywolf, 2019).

16. James Kyung-Jin Lee, "Elegies of Social Life: The Wounded Asian American," *Journal of Race, Ethnicity, and Religion* 3, no. 2.7 (January 2012), 1–21.

17. In a phone call shortly after the publication of her book, Worrall relayed to me that she decided to self-publish after receiving rejection letters from pub-

lishers, with editors telling her that readers didn't want to read "another" breast cancer narrative—despite the lists of breast cancer memoirs that demonstrate the unrelenting demand for such writing: see, e.g., Swapna Krishna, "Breast Cancer Awareness Month: A List of Memoirs," *SheKnows*, July 21, 2015, https://www.she knows.com/entertainment/articles/973507breast-cancer-awareness-month-a-list-of -memoirs. Worrall believes that editors didn't think readers would be interested in an Asian American breast cancer story. I agree with her and, like her, think that editors deeply miscalculated what readers needed to learn from Asian Americans about illness and death.

18. Anatole Broyard, *Intoxicated by My Illness and Other Writings On Life and Death* (New York: Fawcett, 1993), 5.

19. Ibid., 25.

20. Ibid., 44.

21. Ibid., 45.

22. Frank, *Wounded Storyteller*, 27.

23. Ibid.

24. Broyard, *Intoxicated*, 3.

25. Ibid., 7.

26. Henry Louis Gates Jr., "White like Me," *New Yorker*, June 17, 1996, https:// www.newyorker.com/magazine/1996/06/17/white-like-me.

27. Ibid.

28. Broyard, *Intoxicated*, 24.

29. Ibid., 24–25.

30. Constance Valis Hill, *Tap Dancing America: A Cultural History* (New York: Oxford University Press, 2010), 90.

31. Broyard, *Intoxicated*, 12–13.

32. Audre Lorde, *The Cancer Journals: Special Edition* (San Francisco: Aunt Lute, 1997), 28–29.

33. Ibid., 28.

34. Ibid., 29.

35. Ibid., 36.

36. Janice A. Sabin, "How We Fail Black Patients in Pain," Association of American Medical Colleges website, January 6, 2020, https://www.aamc.org/news -insights/how-we-fail-black-patients-pain.

37. Elizabeth Alexander, "'Coming out Blackened and Whole': Fragmentation and Reintegration in Audre Lorde's *Zami* and *The Cancer Journals*," *American Literary History* 6, no. 4 (Winter 1994): 697.

38. Lorde, *Cancer Journals*, 61.

39. Ibid., 10.

40. Cynthia Wu, "Marked Bodies, Marking Time: Reclaiming the Warrior in Audre Lorde's *The Cancer Journals*," *a/b: Auto/Biography Studies* 17, no. 2 (2002): 246.

41. Lorde, *Cancer Journals*, 53.

42. Ibid.

43. Arthur Frank, "Tricksters and Truth Tellers: Narrating Illness in an Age of Authenticity and Appropriation," *Literature and Medicine* 28, no. 2 (Fall 2009): 195.

44. Ho, *Diary*, xl.

45. Ibid., 259.

46. Siddhartha Mukherjee, *Emperor of All Maladies: A Biography of Cancer* (New York: Scribner, 2010), 167–170.

47. Cited in ibid., 180.

48. Ibid., 188.

49. Susan Sontag, *Illness as Metaphor and AIDS and Its Metaphors* (New York: Picador, 2001), 69.

50. Ho's book was followed closely by Brandy Liên Worrall's in 2014, which, as a reminder, was self-published because of the lack of trade interest.

51. Diane C. Fujino, "Introduction: Revolutionary Dreaming and New Dawns," in *Wicked Theory, Naked Practice: The Fred Ho Reader*, edited by Diane C. Fujino (Minneapolis: University of Minnesota Press, 2009), 15–16.

52. Ibid., 7–38.

53. Ho, *Diary*, 255.

54. Ibid., 15.

55. Ibid., 77.

56. Ibid., 240.

57. Ibid., 206, 224.

58. Ibid., 218.

59. Tobin Siebers, *Disability Theory* (Ann Arbor: University of Michigan Press, 2008), 8.

60. Ho, *Diary*, 260.

61. University of California, Irvine, Anti-Cancer Challenge website, n.d., http://www.anti-cancerchallenge.org; Dana-Farber Cancer Institute, "Cracking the Code," video (advertisement), n.d., https://www.ispot.tv/ad/AMD2/dana-farber-cancer-institute-cracking-the-code.

62. This term "care of the self," of course, derives from the third volume of Michel Foucault's *History of Sexuality*, a work that marks a shift in Foucault's thinking from that of biopolitical governmentality to what one might call a bioethics: Michel Foucault, *The History of Sexuality, Volume 3: The Care of the Self*, translated by Robert Hurley (New York: Vintage, 1986); see also Andrew Dilts, "From 'Entrepreneur of the Self' to 'Care of the Self': Neo-liberal Governmentality and Foucault's Ethics," *Foucault Studies* 12 (2011): 130–146.

63. Lorde, *Cancer Journals*, 60.

64. Ibid.

65. Fred Ho, "Beyond Asian American Jazz: My Musical and Political Changes in the Asian American Movement," in Fujino, *Wicked Theory*, 58.

66. S. Lochlann Jain challenges the implied masculinity in the warrior metaphor, even in Lorde, and wonders whether there are other forms of "resistance" to stultifying cultural expectations in living with cancer: S. Lochlann Jain, *Malignant: How Cancer Becomes Us* (Berkeley: University of California Press, 2013), 82.

67. The phrase "wounded storytellers" is from Frank, *Wounded Storyteller*.

68. Worrall, *What Doesn't*, 2.

69. Referenced in Frank, *Wounded Storyteller*, 54.

70. Worrall, *What Doesn't*, 29.

71. Frank, *Wounded Storyteller*, 55.

72. Ibid., 55.

73. Worrall, *What Doesn't*, 57–58.

74. Ibid., 30.

75. Ibid., 212.

76. Ibid., 64.

77. Rob Nixon, *Slow Violence and the Environmentalism of the Poor* (Cambridge, MA: Harvard University Press, 2011); Peter Sills, *Toxic War: The Story of Agent Orange* (Nashville: Vanderbilt University Press, 2014).

78. Worrall, *What Doesn't*, 64–65.

79. Mel Chen, *Animacies: Biopolitics, Racial Meaning, and Queer Affect* (Durham, NC: Duke University Press, 2012), 210–211.

80. Worrall's father died in 2015.

81. "Diagnosis: Damn," *Brandy's Cancer Bash* (blog), July 16, 2007, https://cancerfuckingsucks.blogspot.com/2007/07/diagnosis-damn.html.

82. "Not-so-Dead Arm," *Brandy's Cancer Bash* (blog), August 19, 2008, https://cancerfuckingsucks.blogspot.com/2008/08/not-so-dead-arm.html.

83. Geert Lovink, *Networks without a Cause: A Critique of Social Media* (Malden, MA: Polity, 2011), 100.

84. Ibid., 101.

85. Fred Moten, *Black and Blur* (Durham, NC: Duke University Press, 2017).

86. Jennifer Ann Ho, *Racial Ambiguity in Asian American Culture* (New Brunswick, NJ: Rutgers University Press, 2015), 58.

87. Kimberly McKee, *Disrupting Kinship: Transnational Politics of Korean Adoption in the United States* (Urbana: University of Illinois Press, 2019), 135–144; Eleana J. Kim, *Adopted Territory: Transnational Korean Adoptees and the Politics of Belonging* (Durham, NC: Duke University Press, 2010), 15.

88. Ho, *Racial Ambiguity*, 68.

89. Jennifer Ann Ho, "An Update on Herstories: Breast Cancer Narratives and CounterNarratives," *No F****** Pink Ribbons!* (blog), March 14, 2013, https://nofnpinkribbons.blogspot.com/2013/03/an-update-on-herstories-breast-cancer.html.

90. Jennifer Ann Ho, "Shannon Miller: Ovarian Cancer Survivor," *No F****** Pink Ribbons!* (blog), August 7, 2012, https://nofnpinkribbons.blogspot.com/2012/08/shannon-miller-ovarian-cancer-survivor.html.

91. Ho, *Racial Ambiguity*, 70.

92. Writing under a Pseudonym (Christine Hyung-Oak Lee), "Little Miss Bust," *Jade Park* (blog), September 9, 2006, https://jadepark.wordpress.com/2006/09/09/little-miss-busy.

93. Writing under a Pseudonym (Christine Hyung-Oak Lee), "Brain Brain," *Jade Park* (blog), December 31, 2006, https://jadepark.wordpress.com/2006/12/31/brain-brain.

94. Writing under a Pseudonym (Christine Hyung-Oak Lee), "swimming ideas," *Jade Park* (blog), January 2, 2007, https://jadepark.wordpress.com/2007/01/02/swimming-ideas.

95. Writing under a Pseudonym (Christine Hyung-Oak Lee), "I Stroked Out," *Jade Park* (blog), January 6, 2007, https://jadepark.wordpress.com/2007/01/06/i-stroked-out.

96. Lee, *Tell Me Everything*, 55.

97. Ibid., 38.

98. Ibid., 1.

99. Ibid.

100. Ibid., 2.

101. Ibid., 159.

102. Ibid., 160.

103. Ibid., 73.

104. Ibid., 67.

105. Ibid., 73.

106. Ibid., 102.

107. Ibid., 5.

108. Ibid., 11.

109. Ibid., 84.

110. Frank, *Wounded Storyteller*, 114.

111. Lee, *Tell Me Everything*, 6.

112. Ibid., 87–88.

113. Ibid., 87.

114. Ibid., 46.

115. Ibid., 236.

116. Frank, *Wounded Storyteller*, 129.

117. Lee, *Tell Me Everything*, 199.

118. Ibid., 202.

119. Frank, *Wounded Storyteller*, 142.

120. Lee, *Tell Me Everything*, 216.

121. Ibid., 219.

122. Ibid., 246.

123. Kalanithi, *Breath*, 223.

124. Julie Yip-Williams, *The Unwinding of the Miracle: A Memoir of Life, Death, and Everything That Comes After* (New York: Random House, 2019), 309.

CHAPTER 4

1. Patrick Anderson, *Autobiography of a Disease* (New York: Routledge, 2017), 81.

2. Ibid., ix.

3. Ibid.

4. Ibid., 3.

5. Ibid., 119.

6. Ibid., 220, emphasis added.

7. Ibid., ix.

8. Elaine Scarry, *The Body in Pain: The Making and Unmaking of the World* (New York: Oxford University Press, 1987).

9. Anderson, *Autobiography*, 97.

10. Ibid., 150.

11. S. Lochlann Jain, *Malignant: How Cancer Becomes Us* (Berkeley: University of California Press, 2013), 93.

12. Ibid., 94.

13. Ibid., 4.

14. I wrote this line in early 2019. At the time, I was unaware that, in 2020, a novel coronavirus would leave this ostensible biomedical certainty in tatters.

15. Jain, *Malignant*, 4, emphasis added.

16. Ibid., 5.

17. Ibid., 105.

18. Atul Gawande, *Complications: A Surgeon's Notes on an Imperfect Science* (New York: Picador, 2003).

19. Jain, *Malignant*, 107–108.

20. Ibid., 112.

21. Ibid., 115.

22. Ibid., 117.

23. Ibid., 120.

24. Ibid., 21–22.

25. Ibid., 29.

26. Ibid., 30.

27. Ibid., 216.

28. Cynthia G. Franklin, *Academic Lives: Memoir, Cultural Theory, and the University Today* (Athens: University of Georgia Press, 2009), 2.

29. Ibid., 13.

30. Ibid., 277.

31. This is a clap back to Chapter 2 and Sedgwick's contrast between paranoid and reparative reading. Keep reading this chapter for another rehearsal.

32. Franklin, *Academic Lives*, 276.

33. Ibid., 214.

34. Ibid., 215.

35. Ibid., 216.

36. Ibid., 217.

37. Empathy has profound limits: see Amy Schuman, *Other People's Stories: Entitlement Claims and the Critique of Empathy* (Urbana: University of Illinois Press, 2019). As Schuman puts it, "Empathy describes the sphere of the normal and allows us to imagine what any normal person would do": ibid., 164. What constitutes the empathy of a "normal" person is precisely what Franklin hopes to get at in her critique of the academic memoir, which makes her call for empathy an ironic return to normative affects. Empathy can move you toward interdependence, but it's fraught. We should be open to another affective leans. Try curiosity.

38. Jain, *Malignant*, 46.

39. Ibid., 47.

40. Ibid., 48.

41. Ibid., 216.

42. Ibid., 217.

43. Ibid.

44. Ibid., 223.

45. Ibid.

46. Ibid.

47. Mel Chen, *Animacies: Biopolitics, Racial Meaning, and Queer Affect* (Durham, NC: Duke University Press, 2012), 2.

48. Ibid., 1.

49. Ibid.

50. Ibid., 3.

51. Ibid., 98.

52. Ibid., 189.

53. Ibid., 192.

54. Ibid.

55. Ibid., 196.

56. Ibid., 197.

57. Ibid.

58. Ibid., emphasis added.

59. Ibid., 201.

60. Ibid., 202.

61. Ibid., 203.

62. Here I follow Alison Kafer's careful injunction to explore ways that non-disabled people can "claim crip" not to appropriate but to challenge the poisonous ableist binarisms of disabled-nondisabled or sick-healthy. "To claim crip critically is to recognize the ethical, epistemic, and political responsibilities behind such claims; deconstructing the binary between disabled and able-bodied/able-minded requires more attention to how different bodies/minds are treated differently, not less": Alison Kafer, *Feminist, Queer, Crip* (Bloomington: Indiana University Press, 2013), 13.

63. Chen, *Animacies*, 7.

64. Ibid., 210–211.

65. Jack Halberstam, *The Queer Art of Failure* (Durham, NC: Duke University Press, 2011).

66. Chen, *Animacies*, 218.

67. Ibid.

68. Ibid., 234.

69. Ibid., 237.

70. Lana Lin, *Freud's Jaw and Other Lost Objects: Fractured Subjectivity in the Face of Cancer* (New York: Fordham University Press, 2017), 21.

71. Ibid., 22.

72. Ibid.

73. Ibid.

74. Ibid., 2.

75. Ibid., 155.

76. Ibid.

77. Ibid., 7.

78. Ibid., 13.

79. Ibid., 6.

80. Ibid., 28.

81. Ibid., 39.

82. Ibid., 49.

83. Ibid.

84. Ibid., 73–74.

85. Ibid., 73.

86. Ibid., 59.

87. Ibid., 79.

88. Ibid., 80.

89. Ibid.

90. Lin further explores the community that has emerged from Lorde's narrative about her cancer in a recent film, in which Black women and other women of color (and some white women) read from *The Cancer Journals* and reflect on their own experiences of cancer: Lana Lin, dir., *The Cancer Journals Revisited*, DVD, Women Make Movies, New York, 2018.

91. Lin, *Freud's Jaw*, 81.

92. Ibid.

93. Ibid., 56, 70.

94. Ibid., 152.

95. José Esteban Muñoz, *Disidentifications: Queers of Color and the Performance of Politics* (Minneapolis: University of Minnesota Press, 1999), 12.

96. Lin, *Freud's Jaw*, 153–154.

97. Ibid., 111.

98. Cited in ibid., 102.

99. Ibid., 104.

100. Eve Kosofsky Sedgwick, *Touching Feeling: Affect, Pedagogy, Performativity* (Durham, NC: Duke University Press, 2003), 148–149.

101. Ibid., 149.

102. Ibid.

103. Ibid.

104. Ibid., 150.

105. Lin, *Freud's Jaw*, 110, 112.

106. Arthur Frank, *The Wounded Storyteller: Body, Illness, and Ethics* (Chicago: University of Chicago Press, 1995), 49.

107. Lin, *Freud's Jaw*, 112.

108. Ibid., 113.

109. Leslie T. Hatamiya, *Righting a Wrong: Japanese Americans and the Passage of the Civil Liberties Act of 1988* (Stanford, CA: Stanford University Press, 1993).

110. Reparations would also be the beginning of the United States' finally reckoning with its anti-Black, anti-Indigenous ontology. As an introduction, see Sam Levin, "'This Is All Stolen Land': Native Americans Want More than California's Apology," *The Guardian*, June 21, 2019, https://www.theguardian.com/us-news/2019/jun/20/california-native-americans-governor-apology-reparations; Ta-Nehisi Coates, "The Case for Reparations," *The Atlantic*, June 2014, https://www.theatlantic.com/magazine/archive/2014/06/the-case-for-reparations/361631.

111. Lin, *Freud's Jaw*, 114.

EPILOGUE

1. Lisa Park (Eliza Noh), "Letter to My Sister," in *Making More Waves: New Writing by Asian American Women*, edited by Elaine H. Kim, Lillia V. Villanueva, and Asian Women United of California (Boston: Beacon, 1997), 67.

2. Reuters, "'I Am Not a Virus': France's Asian Community Pushes Back over Xenophobia," *NBC News*, February 4, 2020, https://www.nbcnews.com/news/asian-america/i-am-not-virus-france-s-asian-community-pushes-back-n1129811.

3. Steve Mullis and Heidi Glenn, "New Site Collects Reports of Racism against Asian Americans amid Coronavirus Pandemic," National Public Radio, March 27, 2020, https://www.npr.org/sections/coronavirus-live-updates/2020/03/27/822187627

/new-site-collects-reports-of-anti-asian-american-sentiment-amid-coronavirus-pand; "Stop AAPI Hate," n.d., http://www.asianpacificpolicyandplanningcouncil.org/stop-aapi -hate/?fbclid=IwAR3JVKlK6InoJIVAS2brulW7EGgoVTSPsbiwZxQ16TyRgD4F5V YXI8gTqD0.

4. Katie Rogers, Lara Jakes, and Ana Swanson, "Trump Defense Using 'China Virus' Label, Ignoring Growing Criticism," *New York Times*, March 18, 2020, https://www.nytimes.com/2020/03/18/us/politics/china-virus.html; Lili Loofbourow, "The Real Reason Trump Started Calling the Virus 'Chinese,'" *Slate*, March 21, 2020, https://slate.com/news-and-politics/2020/03/trump-calling-coronavirus -chinese-virus.html; Katie Rogers, "Politicians' Use of 'Wuhan Virus' Starts a Debate Health Experts Wanted to Avoid," *New York Times*, March 10, 2020, https://www .nytimes.com/2020/03/10/us/politics/wuhan-virus.html.

5. "Cancer Statistics," National Cancer Institute, September 25, 2020, https:// www.cancer.gov/about-cancer/understanding/statistics.

6. Esmé Weijun Wang, *The Collected Schizophrenias: Essays* (Minneapolis: Graywolf, 2019), 150.

7. Ibid., 150–151.

8. Ibid., 45.

9. Esmé Weijun Wang, "Chronic Uncertainty: Lessons for a Global Pandemic, from a Permanently Sick Person," TheCut.com, April 3, 2020, https://www.thecut .com/2020/04/how-chronic-illness-prepared-me-for-a-global-pandemic.html.

10. Ibid.

11. Ibid.

12. Mimi Khúc, "Guest Editor's Note," in "Booklet," in "Open in Emergency: A Special Issue on Asian American Mental Health," edited by Mimi Khúc, *Asian American Literary Review* 10, no. 2 (2019): n.p.

13. Johanna Hedva, "Sick Woman Theory," in "DSM II: Asian American Edition," in "Open in Emergency: A Special Issue on Asian American Mental Health," edited by Mimi Khúc, *Asian American Literary Review* 10, no. 2 (2019): 140.

14. Ibid., 146.

15. Khúc, "Guest Editor's Note," n.p.

16. Hedva, "Sick Woman Theory," 147–148.

17. Ibid., 148.

18. Annie McClanahan, *Dead Pledges: Debt, Crisis, and Twenty-first Century Culture* (Palo Alto CA: Stanford University Press, 2016), 197.

19. Or perhaps to engage in radical acts of collective care, as intersectional disability justice activists have been cultivating. "What does it mean to shift our ideas of access and care (whether it's disability, childcare, economic access, or many more) from an individual chore, an unfortunate cost of having an unfortunate body, to a collective responsibility that's maybe even deeply joyful?": Leah Lakshmi Piepzna-Samarasinha, *Care Work: Dreaming Disability Justice* (Vancouver: Arsenal Pulp, 2018), 3.

Bibliography

Adorno, Theodor. "The Essay as Form." *New German Critique*, no. 32 (Spring–Summer 1984): 151–171.

Alam, Eram. "The Care of Foreigners: A History of South Asian Physicians in the United States, 1965–2016." Ph.D. diss., University of Pennsylvania, Philadelphia, 2016.

————. "Cold War Crises: Foreign Medical Graduates Respond to U.S. Doctor Shortages, 1965–1975." *Social History of Medicine* (March 2018): 1–20.

Alexander, Elizabeth. "'Coming out Blackened and Whole': Fragmentation and Reintegration in Audre Lorde's *Zami* and *The Cancer Journals*." *American Literary History* 6, no. 4 (Winter 1994): 695–715.

Anderson, Patrick. *Autobiography of a Disease*. New York: Routledge, 2017.

Anker, Elizabeth S., and Rita Felski, eds. *Critique and Postcritique*. Durham, NC: Duke University Press, 2017.

Asch, Adrienne. "Recognizing Death while Affirming Life: Can End of Life Reform Uphold a Disabled Person's Interest in Continued Life?" *Hastings Center Report* 35, no. 6 (November–December 2005): S31–S36.

Au, Michelle. *This Won't Hurt a Bit (and Other White Lies): My Education in Medicine and Motherhood*. New York: Grand Central, 2011.

Baynton, Douglas. "Disability and the Justification of Inequality in American History." In *The New Disability History: American Perspectives*, edited by Paul Longmore and Lauri Umansky, 33–57. New York: New York University Press, 2001.

Benet-Weiser, Sarah. *AuthenticTM: The Politics of Ambivalence in a Brand Culture*. New York: New York University Press, 2012.

Berlant, Lauren. *Cruel Optimism*. Durham, NC: Duke University Press, 2011.

————. *The Female Complaint: The Unfinished Business of Sentimentality in American Culture*. Durham, NC: Duke University Press, 2008.

Bishop, Jeffrey P. *The Anticipatory Corpse: Medicine, Power, and the Care of the Dying*. South Bend, IN: Notre Dame University, 2011.

Brown, Ivan, Roy I. Brown, and Alice Schippers. "A Quality of Life Perspective on the New Eugenics." *Journal of Policy and Practice in Intellectual Disabilities* 16, no. 2 (June 2019): 121–126.

Broyard, Anatole. *Intoxicated by My Illness and Other Writings on Life and Death*. New York: Fawcett, 1993.

Byock, Ira. *Dying Well: The Prospect for Growth at the End of Life*. New York: Riverhead, 1997.

Chakravorty, Sanjoy, Devesh Kapur, and Nirvikar Singh. *The Other One Percent: Indians in America*. New York: Oxford University Press, 2017.

Chan, Sucheng. "You're Short, Besides!" In *Making Waves: An Anthology of Writings by and about Asian American Women*, edited by Diane Yen-Mai Wong and Asian Women United of California, 265–272. Boston: Beacon, 1989.

Charon, Rita. *Narrative Medicine: Honoring the Stories of Illness*. New York: Oxford University Press, 2008.

Chen, Mel. *Animacies: Biopolitics, Racial Meaning, and Queer Affect*. Durham, NC: Duke University Press, 2012.

Chen, Pauline. *Final Exam: A Surgeon's Reflections on Mortality*. New York: Knopf, 2007.

Cheng, William. *Just Vibrations: The Purpose of Sounding Good*. Ann Arbor: University of Michigan Press, 2016.

Chopra, Deepak. *Ageless Body, Timeless Mind: The Quantum Alternative to Growing Old*. New York: Harmony, 1993.

Clare, Eli. *Brilliant Imperfection: Grappling with Cure*. Durham, NC: Duke University Press, 2017.

Couser, G. Thomas. *Signifying Bodies: Disability in Contemporary Life Writing*. Ann Arbor: University of Michigan Press, 2009.

Danielewicz, Jane. *Contemporary Memoirs in Action: How to Do Things with Memoir*. New York: Palgrave Macmillan, 2018.

Dhingra, Lavina, and Floyd Cheung, eds. *Naming Jhumpa Lahiri: Canons and Controversies*. Lanham, MD: Lexington, 2012.

Diedrich, Lisa. *Treatments: Language, Politics, and the Culture of Illness*. Minneapolis: University of Minnesota Press, 2007.

Dilts, Andrew. "From 'Entrepreneur of the Self' to 'Care of the Self': Neo-liberal Governmentality and Foucault's Ethics." *Foucault Studies* 12 (2011): 130–146.

Dolmage, Jay Timothy. *Disabled upon Arrival: Eugenics, Immigration, and the Construction of Race and Disability*. Columbus: Ohio State University Press, 2018.

Duckworth, Angela. *Grit: The Power of Passion and Perseverance*. New York: Scribner, 2016.

Fan, Christopher T. "Melancholy Transcendence: Ted Chiang and Asian American Postracial Form." *Post45* (November 2014). http://post45.research.yale.edu/2014/11/melancholy-transcendence-ted-chiang-and-asian-american-postracial-form.

Felski, Rita. *The Limits of Critique*. Chicago: University of Chicago Press, 2015.

Fickle, Tara. *The Race Card: From Gaming Technologies to Model Minorities*. New York: New York University Press, 2019.

Foucault, Michel. *The Birth of the Clinic*. Translated by Alan Sheridan Smith. New York: Pantheon, 1973.

———. *The History of Sexuality, Volume 3: The Care of the Self*. Translated by Robert Hurley. New York: Vintage, 1986.

Frank, Arthur. *Letting Stories Breathe: A Socio-Narratology*. Chicago: University of Chicago Press, 2010.

———. "Tricksters and Truth Tellers: Narrating Illness in an Age of Authenticity and Appropriation." *Literature and Medicine* 28, no. 2 (Fall 2009): 185–199.

———. *The Wounded Storyteller: Body, Illness, and Ethics*. Chicago: University of Chicago Press, 1995.

Franklin, Cynthia G. *Academic Lives: Memoir, Cultural Theory, and the University Today*. Athens: University of Georgia Press, 2009.

Fujino, Diane C., ed. *Wicked Theory, Naked Practice: The Fred Ho Reader*. Minneapolis: University of Minnesota Press, 2009.

Gallagher, Nora. *Moonlight Sonata at the Mayo Clinic*. New York: Vintage, 2014.

Garland-Thomson, Rosemarie. "Integrating Disability, Transforming Feminist Theory." *NWSA Journal* 14, no. 3 (Autumn 2002): 1–32.

Gawande, Atul. *Being Mortal: Medicine and What Matters in the End*. New York: Metropolitan, 2014.

———. *Complications: A Surgeon's Notes on an Imperfect Science*. New York: Picador, 2003.

Green, Fiona. "Elizabeth Bishop in Brazil and the *New Yorker*." *Journal of American Studies* 46, no. 4 (2012): 803–829.

Gualtieri, Elena. "The Essay as Form: Virginia Woolf and the Literary Tradition." *Textual Practice* 12, no. 1 (1998): 49–67.

Gupta, Sanjay. *Cheating Death: The Doctors and Medical Miracles That Are Saving Lives against All Odds*. New York: Grand Central Life and Style, 2009.

Halberstam, Jack. *The Queer Art of Failure*. Durham, NC: Duke University Press, 2011.

Hatamiya, Leslie T. *Righting a Wrong: Japanese Americans and the Passage of the Civil Liberties Act of 1988*. Stanford, CA: Stanford University Press, 1993.

Hawkins, Anne Hunsaker. *Reconstructing Illness: Studies in Pathography*. West Lafayette, IN: Purdue University Press, 1998.

Hedva, Johanna. "Sick Woman Theory." In "DSM II: Asian American Edition," in "Open in Emergency: A Special Issue on Asian American Mental Health," edited by Mimi Khúc. *Asian American Literary Review* 10, no. 2 (2019): 142–150.

Held, Virginia. *The Ethics of Care: Personal, Political, and Global.* New York: Oxford University Press, 2007.

Hill, Constance Valis. *Tap Dancing America: A Cultural History.* New York: Oxford University Press, 2010.

Ho, Fred. *Diary of a Radical Cancer Warrior: Fighting Cancer and Capitalism at the Cellular Level.* New York: Skyhorse, 2011.

Ho, Jennifer Ann. *Racial Ambiguity in Asian American Culture.* New Brunswick, NJ: Rutgers University Press, 2015.

Howarth, William. "Oliver Sacks: The Ecology of Writing Science." *Modern Language Studies* 20, no. 4 (Autumn 1990): 103–120.

Hsu, Madeline Y. *The Good Immigrants: How the Yellow Peril Became the Model Minority.* Princeton, NJ: Princeton University Press, 2015.

Hull, Andrew John. "Fictional Father? Oliver Sacks and the Revalidation of Pathography." *Medical Humanities* 39 (2013): 105–114.

"An Introduction to *The New Yorker.*" In *Twentieth-Century Literary Criticism*, vol. 58, edited by Jennifer Gariepy, 274–295. Detroit: Gale, 1995. http://link.gale group.com/apps/doc/GOLOCV654144738/LCO?u=univca20&sid=LCO&xid =c30a3b78.

Irvine, Craig. "The Other Side of Silence: Levinas, Medicine, and Literature." *Literature and Medicine* 24, no. 1 (February 2005): 8–18.

Iwamura, Jane. *Virtual Orientalism: Asian Religions and American Popular Culture.* New York: Oxford University Press, 2011.

Jain, S. Lochlann. *Malignant: How Cancer Becomes Us.* Berkeley: University of California Press, 2013.

Jauhar, Sandeep. *Intern: A Doctor's Initiation.* New York: Farrar, Straus and Giroux, 2007.

Jurecic, Ann. *Illness as Narrative.* Pittsburgh: University of Pittsburgh Press, 2012.

Kafer, Alison. *Feminist, Queer, Crip.* Bloomington: Indiana University Press, 2013.

Kalanithi, Paul. *When Breath Becomes Air.* New York: Random House, 2016.

Khúc, Mimi. "Guest Editor's Note." In "Booklet," in "Open in Emergency: A Special Issue on Asian American Mental Health," edited by Mimi Khúc. *Asian American Literary Review* 10, no. 2 (2019): n.p.

Kim, Claire Jean. "The Racial Triangulation of Asian Americans." *Politics and Society* 27, no. 1 (1999): 105–138.

Kim, Eleana J. *Adopted Territory: Transnational Korean Adoptees and the Politics of Belonging.* Durham, NC: Duke University Press, 2010.

Kim, Eunjung. *Curative Violence: Rehabilitating Disability, Gender, and Sexuality in Modern Korea.* Durham, NC: Duke University Press, 2017.

Kim, Ronyoung. *Clay Walls.* Sag Harbor, NY: Permanent, 1987.

Kusnetz, Ella. "The Soul of Oliver Sacks." *Massachusetts Review* 33, no. 2 (Summer 1992): 175–198.

Lahiri, Jhumpa. *In Other Words*. Translated by Ann Goldstein. New York: Knopf, 2016.

———. *The Namesake*. New York: Houghton Mifflin, 2003.

———. "Teach Yourself Italian." *New Yorker*, vol. 91, no. 39, December 7, 2015, 30–36. https://www.newyorker.com/magazine/2015/12/07/teach-yourself-italian.

Lakshmi, Padma. *Love, Loss, and What We Ate: A Memoir*. New York: Ecco, 2016.

Latour, Bruno. "Why Has Critique Run Out of Steam? From Matters of Fact to Matters of Concern." *Critical Inquiry* 30 (2004): 225–248.

Lee, Christine Hyung-Oak. *Tell Me Everything You Don't Remember: The Stroke That Changed My Life*. New York: Ecco, 2017.

Lee, James Kyung-Jin. "Elegies of Social Life: The Wounded Asian American." *Journal of Race, Ethnicity, and Religion* 3, no. 2.7 (January 2012): 1–21.

Lee, Jennifer, and Min Zhou. *The Asian American Achievement Paradox*. New York: Russell Sage Foundation, 2015.

Lee, Rachel C. *The Exquisite Corpse of Asian America: Biopolitics, Biosociality, and Posthuman Ecologies*. New York: New York University Press, 2014.

Lin, Lana, dir. *The Cancer Journals Revisited*. DVD. Women Make Movies, New York, 2018.

———. *Freud's Jaw and Other Lost Objects: Fractured Subjectivity in the Face of Cancer*. New York: Fordham University Press, 2017.

Lorde, Audre. *The Cancer Journals: Special Edition*. San Francisco: Aunt Lute, 1997.

Lovink, Geert. *Networks without a Cause: A Critique of Social Media*. Malden, MA: Polity, 2011.

Lukács, György. *Soul and Form*. Edited by John T. Sanders and Katie Terazakis. Translated by Anna Bostock. New York: Columbia University Press, 2010.

Mack, Katherine, and Jonathan Alexander. "The Ethics of Memoir: *Ethos* in Uptake." *Rhetoric Society Quarterly* 49, no. 1 (2019): 49–70.

Marini, Irmo. "Cross-Cultural Counseling Issues of Males Who Sustain a Disability." In *The Psychological and Social Impact of Illness and Disability*, 6th ed., edited by Irmo Marini and Mark Stebnicki, 151–164. New York: Springer, 2012.

McClanahan, Annie. *Dead Pledges: Debt, Crisis, and Twenty-first Century Culture*. Palo Alto, CA: Stanford University Press, 2016.

McGurl, Mark. *The Program Era: Postwar Fiction and the Rise of Creative Writing*. Cambridge, MA: Harvard University Press, 2011.

McKee, Kimberly D. *Disrupting Kinship: Transnational Politics of Korean Adoption in the United States*. Urbana: University of Illinois Press, 2019.

Moten, Fred. *Black and Blur*. Durham, NC: Duke University Press, 2017.

Mukherjee, Siddhartha. *Emperor of All Maladies: A Biography of Cancer*. New York: Scribner, 2010.

————. *Gene: An Intimate History*. New York: Scribner, 2016.

Mullan, Fitzhugh. "The Metrics of the Physician Brain Drain." *New England Journal of Medicine* 353 (2005): 1810–1818.

Muñoz, José Esteban. *Disidentifications: Queers of Color and the Performance of Politics*. Minneapolis: University of Minnesota Press, 1999.

Ninh, erin Khuê. *Ingratitude: The Debt-Bound Daughter in Asian American Literature*. New York: New York University Press, 2009.

Nixon, Rob. *Slow Violence and the Environmentalism of the Poor*. Cambridge, MA: Harvard University Press, 2011.

Nuland, Sherwin. *How We Die: Reflections on Life's Final Chapter*. New York: Knopf, 1994.

Ofri, Danielle. *What Patients Say, What Doctors Hear*. New York: Beacon, 2017.

Osajima, Keith. "Asian Americans as the Model Minority: An Analysis of the Popular Press Image in the 1960s and 1980s." In *Reflections on Shattered Windows: Promises and Prospects for Asian American Studies*, edited by Gary Okihiro, 165–174. Pullman: Washington State University Press, 1988.

Park, Lisa (Eliza Noh). "Letter to My Sister." In *Making More Waves: New Writing by Asian American Women*, edited by Elaine H. Kim, Lillia V. Villanueva, and Asian Women United of California, 65–71. Boston: Beacon, 1997.

Pennycook, Gordon, James Allan Cheyne, Nathaniel Barr, Derek J. Koehler, and Jonathan A. Fugelsang. "On the Reception and Deception of Pseudo-Profound Bullshit." *Judgment and Decision Making* 10, no. 6 (November 2015): 549–563.

Piepzna-Samarasinha, Leah Lakshmi. *Care Work: Dreaming Disability Justice*. Vancouver: Arsenal Pulp, 2018.

Poirier, Suzanne. *Doctors in the Making: Memoirs and Medical Education*. Kindle ed. Iowa City: University of Iowa Press, 2009.

Prashad, Vijay. *The Karma of Brown Folk*. Minneapolis: University of Minnesota Press, 2000.

Prentice, Rachel. *Bodies in Formation: An Ethnography of Anatomy and Surgery Education*. Durham, NC: Duke University Press, 2013.

Price, Margaret. "The Bodymind Problem and the Possibilities of Pain." *Hypatia* 30, no. 1 (Winter 2015): 268–284.

Puri, Sunita. *That Good Night: Life and Medicine in the Eleventh Hour*. New York: Viking, 2019.

Rangaswamy, Padma. *Namasté America: Indian Immigrants in an American Metropolis*. University Park: Pennsylvania State University Press, 2000.

Robbins, Bruce. "Not So Well Attached." *PMLA* 132, no. 2 (2017), 371–376.

Sacks, Oliver. *An Anthropologist on Mars: Seven Paradoxical Tales*. New York: Knopf, 1995.

————. *On the Move: A Life*. New York: Knopf, 2015.

Scarry, Elaine. *The Body in Pain: The Making and Unmaking of the World*. New York: Oxford University Press, 1987.

Schuman, Amy. *Other People's Stories: Entitlement Claims and the Critique of Empathy.* Urbana: University of Illinois Press, 2019.

Sedgwick, Eve Kosofsky. *Touching Feeling: Affect, Pedagogy, Performativity.* Durham, NC: Duke University Press, 2003.

Siebers, Tobin. "Disability in Theory: From Social Constructionism to the New Realism of the Body." In *The Disability Studies Reader*, 2d ed., edited by Lennard J. Davis, 173–184. New York: Routledge, 2006.

———. *Disability Theory.* Ann Arbor: University of Michigan Press, 2008.

Sills, Peter. *Toxic War: The Story of Agent Orange.* Nashville: Vanderbilt University Press, 2014.

Singh, Prabhjot. *Dying and Living in the Neighborhood: A Street-Level View of America's Healthcare Promise.* Baltimore: Johns Hopkins University Press, 2016.

Snyder, Sharon L., and David T. Mitchell. *Cultural Locations of Disability.* Chicago: University of Chicago Press, 2005.

Song, Min Hyoung. "The Children of 1965: Allegory, Postmodernism, and Jhumpa Lahiri's *The Namesake.*" *Twentieth-Century Literature* 53, no. 3 (Fall 2007): 345–370.

———. *The Children of 1965: On Writing, and Not Writing, as an Asian American.* Durham, NC: Duke University Press, 2013.

Sontag, Susan. *Illness as Metaphor and AIDS and Its Metaphors.* New York: Picador, 2001.

Srikanth, Rajini. "Ethnic Outsider as the Ultimate Insider: The Paradox of Verghese's 'My Own Country.'" *MELUS* 29, nos. 3–4 (Autumn–Winter 2004): 433–450.

Tweedy, Damon. *Black Man in a White Coat.* New York: Picador, 2015.

Verghese, Abraham. *My Own Country: A Doctor's Story of a Town and Its People in the Age of AIDS.* New York: Simon and Schuster, 1994.

Wailoo, Keith. *How Cancer Crossed the Color Line.* New York: Oxford University Press, 2011.

Wang, Esmé Weijun. *The Collected Schizophrenias: Essays.* Minneapolis: Graywolf, 2019.

Wong, Paul, Chienping Faith Lai, Richard Nagasawa, and Tieming Lin. "Asian Americans as a Model Minority: Self-Perceptions and Perceptions by Other Racial Groups." *Sociological Perspectives* 41, no. 1 (1998): 95–118.

Worrall, Brandy Liên. *What Doesn't Kill Us.* Vancouver: Rabbit Fool, 2014.

Wu, Cynthia. *Chang and Eng Reconnected: The Original Siamese Twins in American Culture.* Philadelphia: Temple University Press, 2012.

———. "Marked Bodies, Marking Time: Reclaiming the Warrior in Audre Lorde's *The Cancer Journals.*" *a/b: Auto/Biography Studies* 17, no. 2 (2002): 245–261.

Wu, Ellen D. *The Color of Success: Asian Americans and the Origins of the Model Minority.* Princeton, NJ: Princeton University Press, 2013.

Yamamoto, Hisaye. "Las Vegas Charley." In *Seventeen Syllables and Other Stories*, 70–85. New Brunswick, NJ: Rutgers University Press, 2001.

Yip-Williams, Julie. *The Unwinding of the Miracle: A Memoir of Life, Death, and Everything That Comes After*. New York: Random House, 2019.

Youn, Anthony, with Alan Eisenstock. *In Stitches: A Memoir*. New York: Gallery, 2011.

Young, Michelle. *What Patients Taught Me: A Medical Student's Journey*. Seattle: Sasquatch, 2007.

Index

Abani, Chris, 124

ableism: activism and, 108–110; Asian American bodies and, 176n29; in disability studies, 37, 147, 182n73; Hart-Celler Act and, 42, 65; humanness and, 42, 143; in illness memoirs, 18; model minority discourse and, 6, 8, 10–11, 166; scholarly engagement with, 147–148

activism, 137; ableism and, 8, 108–110; anti-Asian violence, response to, 163–164; disability, 180n36, 196n19; of Fred Ho, 17, 108–110

Adorno, Theodor, 48–49, 56

Affordable Care Act, 56

Agamben, Giorgio, 176n29

Alam, Eram, 32–33, 35, 178n14

Alexander, Elizabeth, 103, 148–149

allopathic medicine, 18, 34, 36, 108–109

American exceptionalism, 33

American Medical Association (AMA), 33, 178n14

Americanness: Asian Americans and, 163; as racism, 162

Anderson, Patrick, 127–129, 131–132

Animacies (Mel Chen), 141–149; animacy in, 146–147, 149; coexistence in, 148–149; disability politics in, 142; humanness in, 142–143; interdependency in, 146; intimacy in, 145–147; language in, 147; toxicity in, 141, 144–149, 151, 160

Arendt, Hannah, 48

Asian adoption, 115–116

Asian Americanness, 91, 113

Asian Americans: in the arts and humanities, 45; assimilation of, 163; identity of, 65, 82, 83–84, 163; illness and, 5–6, 120–121; invisibility of, 174n9; as model minorities, 64, 119; self-perceptions of, 175n14; stereotypes of, 66–67; success frame of, 3, 161; visibility of, 168, 174n9. *See also* bodies, Asian American; model minorities; model minority discourse; South Asian Americans

Asian American studies, 164; ableism and, 8; Asian American bodies in, 8–9; critique of model minority discourse, 7–8; disability studies and, 8–9

assimilation: of Asian Americans, 9, 163; model minority discourse and, 10, 163; in *The Namesake*, 28–29; pedagogy of, 28–29, 30

Au, Michelle: as model minority, 67; *This Won't Hurt a Bit*, 11, 66–71, 75–76, 79. See also *This Won't Hurt a Bit* (Au)

autism, 47

Autobiography of a Disease (Anderson), 127–129; multiple subjectivities in, 129; race and gender in, 131–132

autoethnography, 43, 127

Ayurvedic medicine, 34–35, 36

Baldwin, James, 48

Barazanji, Zeyad, 38

James Kyung-Jin Lee is an Associate Professor of Asian American Studies and English and Director of the Center for Medical Humanities at the University of California, Irvine. He is the author of *Urban Triage: Race and the Fictions of Multiculturalism*.

www.ingramcontent.com/pod-product-compliance
Lightning Source LLC
Chambersburg PA
CBHW022356280326
41935CB00007B/205